BODY-FLOW

FREEDOM FROM FEAR-REACTIVITY

By **Scott Sonnon**

BODY-FLOW:

FREEDOM FROM FEAR-REACTIVITY

For information address:
RMAX.tv Productions
P.O. Box 501388
Atlanta, GA 31150
Website: www.RMAX.tv
Email comments and questions to: info@RMAX.tv

FIRST EDITION

CREDITS:

Cover Art Design:	Barry Crain
Editing:	Michael Gannon, Phil Elmore
Photography:	Brad Kenyon, Aurora Films, LLC www.aurorafilms.com

ISBN: 0-9717949-3-6

Disclaimer: The information in this book is presented in good faith, but no warranty is given, nor results guaranteed. Since we have no control over physical conditions surrounding the application of information in this book the author and publisher disclaim any liability for untoward results including (but not limited) any injuries or damages arising out of any person's attempt to rely upon any information herein contained. The exercises described in this book are for information purposes, and may be too strenuous or even dangerous for some people. The reader should consult a physician before starting clubbells or any other exercise programs.

IMPORTANT: Please be sure to thoroughly read the instructions for all exercises in this book, paying particular attention to all cautions and warnings shown for clubbells to ensure their proper and safe use.

ABOUT THE AUTHOR

USA National Coach several times over, Scott Sonnon became an internationally-ranked champion in the fighting sport of SAMBO, a specialized form of grappling which became the 2nd style of international submission fighting. This unique sport has been recognized by the International Olympic Committee for consideration as an Olympic sport. Coach Sonnon served as the International Category Referee in the sport, as well as the International Combat SAMBO Chairman for the Fédération Internationale Amateur de SAMBO (FIAS), the international governing body.

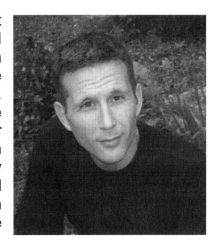

Due to his international record and his contributions to the growth of the sport, Coach Sonnon received the *Distinguished Master of Sport in SAMBO*, the highest award that can be earned. Having trained many world champions in various sports such as kickboxing, sambo, judo and jiujitsu, he has been inducted into the *International Martial Arts Hall of Fame* three times as a result of his dedication to improving the lives of others through physical culture.

To bring the secrets of his training to the American public, he co-founded RMAX.tv Productions with Nikolay Travkin. The company's mission is to help you become *more prepared than the challenges you'll face*. Scott Sonnon is the Head Coach of the *Life Enhancement Solutions*™ Department at RMAX.tv Productions.

Inadvertantly, a decade ago at the time of this book, Scott Sonnon created a new industry: *Life Enhancement Solutions*™. He discovered that although groups and individuals requested his services across several industries, his coaching pedagogy remained constant, though tailored to the interpretation of the venue. He discovered that a dedication to organic improvement of the group and the individual within the group proved to be paramount to any field or discipline in which he was asked to provide guidance.

As a result, Coach Sonnon has created over 50 videos and books on various aspects of peak performance psychology, sports performance enhancement, fitness and martial arts. He continues to be invited worldwide to give talks to Fortune 500 companies, Professional Sports Teams, Military Units, Police Departments, Actor's Guilds, Professional Health Care Institutions and Universities.

Despite his high in-demand status, he spends as much of his time as possible now in what he calls his most important vocation: adventuring with family and friends. As he often quotes Helen Keller, *"Life is either a daring adventure, or nothing at all."*

DEDICATION

We will be lone travelers, but we journey up the same Mountain..
We will face ominous challenges, but we do so as an united front.
We will encounter our greatest fears, but we do so for our common welfare.
We will face failure, but we will overcome them enthusiastically for a Higher Cause...
And thereby we can never fail.

Stay the course.

We are all alone in this... together.

- Coach Sonnon

PROLOGUE

By Ken Harper

Now and then we encounter people who make a difference in our lives and, in turn, the lives of others. Usually they make their impact through their work, especially if it causes us to do something that makes us healthier, richer, more perceptive, more knowledgeable, etc. In other words, we *feel* better than we did before they (and/or their work) entered our lives. That has been my experience ever since I met Coach Sonnon.

I "met" Coach Sonnon through the video encyclopedia he produced entitled <u>*Zdorovye – The Russian Natural Fitness System*</u>, a word that I'm told means "health" in Russian. *Zdorovye* is a compendium of movements coordinated with breathing regimens – I hesitate to say "exercise" – because of the word's connotations – that are based on Russian health practices. I later learned from Nikolay Travkin, a Russian émigré and Coach Sonnon's business partner, that the movements found in the four-part video encyclopedia *Zdorovye* are actually a collection of different movements that Coach Sonnon encountered at different times in his training with former Soviet Olympics sports trainers and Russian Special Forces (*Spetznaz*). In other words, Coach Sonnon was the "synthesist" and composer, if you will, of *Zdorovye*. It's not a program or curriculum you'd find if you visited Russia today.

As someone who, chronologically, was classified as "middle aged" (51 at the time), my days as an athlete and soldier were well behind me. Ditto most of the hair on my head. I could definitely see how *Zdorovye* might fit into my immediate future.

Zdorovye not only eliminated the stiffness and soreness, but it opened up parts of my body that I'm not sure I'd ever been aware of. As a matter of fact, the practice of *Zdorovye* made me *feel* as I'd never felt before. Doing the *Zdorovye* movements in the morning, I had energy the like and kind I hadn't felt in decades – if then.

As a practitioner of Yoga, Tai Chi and Qigong, I knew that certain movements could open up "energy channels," and as a former jogger, I was also extremely familiar with "runner's high," when the body releases *endorphins*, or natural pain-killers, after you've run for an extended period, usually a half hour or more. The feeling from performing *Zdorovye* was all of that and more.

What was really unique about Coach Sonnon's instructional methods on the tapes was his insistence that these moves were simply building blocks for the viewers to learn in order to compose their own "routines," or to put different movements together (along with the coordinated breathing) in ways that were appropriate for us. In other words, you become your own teacher. Or to put it another way, your body becomes its own instructor.

I went further with Coach Sonnon's instructional materials and obtained the <u>*Grappler's Toolbox (GTB)*</u>, again, a three-volume video "encyclopedia" of movements to help you become more proficient at "grappling" by developing enhanced joint strength and mobility, as well as something Coach Sonnon called "Stored Elastic Energy," which occurs when tendons are properly loaded and unloaded by various body movements. I had been a wrestler in high school, back in the Paleolithic Period of the 1960s, and later attended graduate school at the University of Iowa when the legendary Dan Gable produced indomitable individuals and teams.

As a former football player and an aspiring amateur boxer in the Army until I got my bell rung by the middleweight champion of the 82nd Airborne Division, I knew from experience that the sport of wrestling – real wrestling, not the WWE variety – produced superbly conditioned athletes. The *Grapplers Toolbox* featured many movements that were "advanced" versions of the *Zdorovye* movements, not surprising because, as I learned, the *GTB* was based on, once again, training regimens Coach Sonnon had encountered during his "extended education" in the former Soviet Union. *GTB*, in turn, had *Zdorovye* as its foundation.

Furthermore, because of the acrobatic, gymnastic nature of some of the movements taught in *GTB*, I have come perilously close to learning how to "break dance." (Imagine how embarrassing it might be for my teenage daughter to have her 53-year old father spinning on his back or twirling on his forearms and wrists or doing walking handstands to rap music.) It turns out that some of the *GTB/Zdorovye* movements have their origins in ancient Russian and Slavic folk dance, one of which is called "Break-Down Happy Dance." If you have any doubts about the acrobatic and gymnastic qualities of Russian folk dances, check out a performance of Cossack dancers and then try squatting and kicking "simultaneously" with your arms clasped in front of your chest!♦

So add agility, gymnastics, acrobatics, flexibility, and mobility into the strength endurance mix and you've almost got about half the picture of what you're dealing with when go on an extended "educational" program with Coach Sonnon.

Coach Sonnon has produced a series of videos designed to help martial artists and those involved in the combat arts – and there is more than a semantic difference between the two – better achieve their potential regardless of their "game." In fact, I'm embarrassed to say how long it took me to realize this, but just as with the *Zdorovye* Encyclopedia and *Grapplers Toolbox*, the martial arts/combat arts/self-defense tapes are all designed to help *you teach yourself how to create your own 'style,' based on your unique body and mind AND the situation you find yourself in.*

Coach Sonnon would probably cringe to find the word "style" in the sentence above, but I include it because it's the way I've been programmed to think about martial arts and/or self-defense: i.e., that we need to learn or know some kind of *style* before we go out in the so-called 'real world' and deal with absolutely unique circumstances. Face it: if you've learned a certain school of martial art or self-defense – i.e., karate, Tae-kwon-do, etc. -- the only time you'll ever encounter someone else who will do something in a way you've *learned to respond to is if you've both learned the same 'school' or style* and it will most likely be a sporting event, not a matter of life or death or somewhere in between.

♦ Anyone thinking about learning Capoeira, the popular Brazilian martial arts/dance form, might want to spend some time with Coach Sonnon.

In my 40s, I dabbled in various martial arts practices – Karate, Tae-kwon-do, Pa-kua-chang, Tai-chi, and Aikido. My motivation was varied: I wanted to be able to protect my family, not to mention myself, and I was intrigued by the graceful movements as well as the elements of self-control – the unity of mind and body. I was a serious practitioner of meditation and always marveled at how "unified" I could be in the 20 minutes to half-hour I meditated in the early morning or late night, but I was dismayed at the "disunity" I displayed during those in-between times, despite my diurnal and nocturnal incantations to "be present in the moment." I was usually just "presently" pissed off, stressed, or frightened – with vary degrees of "out of control-ness."

Because of my high-pressure, high-tech job, I had difficulty making the time to afford classes taught by various "masters," and had little patience with their lieutenants who were usually excellent at teaching rote forms but weren't authorized to answer questions about theory or the science behind the forms, etc. Given my peculiar schedule and nagging curiosity for more resources and information, it was much easier to learn from basic moves from tapes – *kata* in the case of Karate, *poomse* for Tae-kwon-do, and the short and long-forms of different families of Tai-chi. As for theory, there were books.

I spent a small fortune on books and tapes, and invested the most precious commodity of the self-employed: time (In 1998 I started my own business.)

The net effect of what I was learning and doing – or not learning and not being able to do – was brought home early one Saturday morning when I took our then 3-year-old daughter to the Portland Zoo and we became bystanders in a violent incident in the parking lot involving three men. Two men pursued a third, over and around parked cars, occasionally catching him, and then they engaged in hand-to-hand fighting, punching, tackling, grappling, kicking, head butting and biting. I recall vividly one of the men screaming, "You bit me! You broke my finger!" And then the third guy would escape, and his pursuers would start all over again. This went on for maybe five minutes until they ran out of the parking lot and my daughter and I entered the Zoo.

I later learned the while watching the news that a convict had escaped at the Portland Zoo from detectives who suspected him of being involved in a series of burglaries not far from where I lived. A police drawing of the suspect looked like the man being pursued in the parking lot.

Although I'd volunteered for the Special Forces while I was in Vietnam, and worked on occasion with them and the CIA, my military training in the late 1960s and the 11 months and 11 days I spent "over there" from 1970-71, left me comically un-armed. For a variety of reasons, I don't own a gun, nor would I have thought to carry one with me to the Portland Zoo. (I'm not a hunter either, especially of caged critters.)

What really struck me about the Katzenjammer Kids scene my daughter and I watched in the Portland Zoo parking lot that morning was how *paralyzed* I was by my inability to figure out what to do, and how best to protect my daughter when the thundering herd came our way or even to make our way stealthily to the nearest phone to call the police who were, of course, already on the scene. The sight of grown men punching, kicking, grappling, and gouging each other – and the possibility of being drawn into it – was frightening. There's no other word for it. Worse, not only was it frightening, but the fear kept me from doing anything other than standing behind a tree with my daughter and watching to see how close they'd get to us. At one point, they all raced past us and, five yards away, the later identified convict banged off a chain-linked fence and then joked and assailed his pursuers until he got away from them again. *Be still, my beating heart.*

When she asked me what the men were doing, I caught my breath and said, "Playing chase."

That same sense of astonishment occurred last week at a "Potluck" Christmas dinner for Portland's homeless individuals and families. A skinny, bearded young man became incensed when a "Potluck Dinner Person" asked him respectfully and repeatedly to leave. (I don't know why.) Flailing his arms, telling the Potluck Dinner Person – a woman with her hands clasped in front of her in the classic prayer position – in no uncertain terms what she could do with herself and what he would do to her if she put her hands on him again, he appeared to be on the verge of violence. There were no police and, as far as I could see, no "security personnel."

I told my now 15-year-old daughter and 12-year-old son to go join their mother, who was getting instructions on what we needed to do as part of the clean-up crew. For my part, I began doing "performance breathing," something I'd learned from Scott to unify body in mind in preparation for "flow state," calculating what I might do if the disturbed young man pulled a knife or used a fork or any one of several poles (holding Christmas garlands) as a weapon to assault the Pot Luck Dinner Person. He didn't.

I have no idea what would have happened if the young man at the Potluck Christmas Dinner had turned violent, but, unlike the time at the Zoo, this time I was prepared to respond with "eyes wide open," cognizant of him as well as the surroundings.

The difference between the Portland Zoo Parking Lot and the Christmas Potluck Dinner was the time I'd invested in Coach Sonnon's various "martial arts" courses and the practice I'd put into planning – if only thinking about – how to deal with unexpected violence. Thich Nhat Hanh, a Vietnamese Buddhist monk I know and revere, who was nominated for the Nobel Peace Prize by Martin Luther King, Jr. for his work during the Vietnam War and afterwards with the boat people and the pirates who ravaged them, advises us to practice in all situations: "clear seeing and calm abiding." This is sometimes easier said than done – **except if you have an idea of how to practice the doing rather than just the saying.** Coach Sonnon's version of the **doing** rather than just the saying is articulated in *Flow Fighting*, a Peak Performance Training video and audio recording from RMAX.tv Productions.

Basically, it's the ability to be fully present in the moment, body and mind acting as a unity. Thomas Hanna, a physical therapist and one of Coach Sonnon's mentors who is cited early in **Body-Flow**, was himself a student of Israeli judoka and research physicist Moshe Feldenkrais. Hanna points out in *Somatics* and other books that it is impossible for humans to think without involving their bodies. In other words, thoughts have physical counterparts and effects.

The reverse is also true: read *The Mind and the Brain: Neuroplasticity and the Power of Mental Force* by Jeffrey M. Schwartz (M.D.), and Sharon Begley. Schwartz, a UCLA psychiatrist and mindfulness practitioner, describes and documents "experiments" done with a wide variety of individuals, showing that "thinking" caused certain areas of the

h

brain to grow as new functionalities and capabilities were added or increased through practice, and that mindfulness plus conscious thought could produce physical actions (or inactions) previously thought impossible by the practitioners. Bodies in motion are "conscious" bodies. The question is how conscious and to what effect? The answer depends on the kinds of practice you engage in. **The practices described in _Body-Flow_ will enhance the process and the results**.

This ability to be "fully present in the moment," or, if you prefer, **_Body-Flow_**, which I attribute largely to Coach Sonnon's teaching me to teach myself, has also been of tremendous benefit in dealing with business setbacks (yes, the economic _downturn_ is real, and if or when it turns down on you, you'll discover how quickly your unity – your body and mind acting together – are tested). The ability to be fully present has also been helpful in dealing with the occasional, unexpected seizures my son suffers from as a by-product of, again, unexpected brain surgery when he was 19 months old.

These petit mal seizures were dormant for almost 11 years, until the Saturday after September 11th – that September 11th – when, at the breakfast table with two friends who'd spent the night, he made a groaning sound, rolled his eyes, and swooned, pitching forward into my arms. I cleared his tongue from his throat (unnecessarily, it turned out), and told my panicked wife to call "9-1-1" and then I just held him and told him in comforting tones to "relax" and that he would be all right, and within less than a minute he was. Fortunately.

Unfortunately, I'm sure we can all come up with examples that are far beyond what I've just described. For me, a frequent flyer on business, and who was scheduled to take a non-stop Washington, D.C., to San Jose, CA flight literally a week before September 11th, one of the most astonishing stories of that tragic day was the group on Flight 93 who decided to counter-attack the terrorists and kept that plane from reaching a target, although their efforts cost them their lives. According to published reports, the group that counter-attacked consisted of a small number of men with martial arts training.

I've often asked myself: what would I have done?

As I think of the pain we all encounter and learn to endure as part of our life's path, I struggle to think of non-pharmaceutical ways not simply to "deal" with them, but to transform the energy locked up by various muscular contractions and resulting skeletal deformations caused by habitual reactions (rather than responses) to "life." (If you're interested in a thorough-going discussion of this, try Thomas Hanna's _Somatic_, which is based, in part, on his education at the hands – literally – of Moshe Feldenkrais, an Israeli judoka and research physicist, whose practice of Structural Integration was instrumental in showing the "unity" of body and mind and simple practices that could be used by people with all sorts of conditions ranging from cerebral palsy to post-exercise stiffness to not simply relieve the tension but bring 'unity' to the body experiencing the mind's thoughts.)

We know that in the United States alone more than 35 million people suffer from arthritis, and that, within the "business world," over 60% of workers, most of them white collar, suffer from "bad backs." On June 23, 2002, the New York Times reported "about 25 percent of adult Americans are thought to live with chronic pain; about 60 percent of them are women." The most common chronic pain conditions for women were listed as:

Tension Headaches

Migraines

Temporomandibular disorders (problems with the jaw joints or muscles)

Fybromyalgia ("fatigue and widespread aches in muscles or joints')

Arthritis

Endometriosis

Back pain

Irritable bowel syndrome

Carpal tunnel syndrome

As you'll read in **Body-Flow**, <u>**many of these conditions have been alleviated or entirely abated by Zdorovye and related health practices**</u>. Simple body movements – and the triggering thoughts – that we are all capable of, if only we'll do it.

Finally, for you hardcore strength enthusiasts, Coach Sonnon references material from _Clubbell Training for Circular Strength_, his book he published this past year. _Circular Strength Training_ is largely for those athletes, martial artists, and combat artists who need to develop the kind of functional strength required by most sports and athletic contests: mainly, _strength while in dynamic motion_. I.e., the kind of strength pitchers need when throwing a baseball, or tennis players require when serving and volleying, and quarterbacks need when letting fly a pass, and boxers require when punching or Judokas, wrestlers or Sambo players need when throwing an opponent. (To get the background on how and why Coach Sonnon developed _Circular Strength Training_, I suggest you read the book.)

I think of Coach Sonnon as one of those rare individuals described in the Bible as a "paraclete," or a helper. Specifically, someone who helps others help themselves, teaching them to fish (and, to extend the metaphor, even how to cook it) rather than simply supplying the fish.

So, if it isn't already apparent, I think Coach Sonnon and **Body-Flow**, in particular, has something to offer everyone. That's right – _everyone_. I once worked for a very successful company (at that time) where the management philosophy and company culture was to "speak with facts." I am not exaggerating when I say that anyone can learn something from **Body-Flow** to make himself or herself healthier, more knowledge, more fit, stronger, leaner, faster, etc.

You might even teach yourself to be happy, regardless of the circumstances you find yourself in. But to do that you'll have to do something: for starters, read the book and then practice, practice, and practice some more.

Ken Harper
Beaverton, Oregon
January 2002

k

All movement balances stability and mobility…The most constant force is gravity…friction and reaction…**Zero Position**…*Zeno's Paradox*…**Body-Flow** is always moving *through* positions… Position => Opposition => Composition… technique is absent…Composition of Forces… movements determine your thoughts

Efficiently integrate your Breathing, Movement and Structure…Acquisition of effective and efficient movement strategies…*Functional Neuromuscular Conditioning*…imposing specific agility, coordination, and balance demands…a vehicle for producing great increases…Becoming aware of the basics

Biomechanical Exercise™ as *practice*…bodyweight exercise as *training*…the grace and poise of *Biomechanical Exercise™* is not so easy…*Biomechanical Exercise™* augments the quality of your movement

Your core determines the success, health and strength of your performance…Recent research…positive health and performance impact…the crux of the matter…integrate your breathing, movement and structure in all your activities

Natural breathing methods that facilitate and augment your natural talent…Oxygen Debt…anaerobic processes…*Performance Breathing*…the three levels of breathing…*2nd Wind*…Mental Toughness…Matter over Mind…Breath Holding…Hypoxic versus Hypercapnic…*Hyperventilation Feedback Loop*…Over-Breathing…*Power Breathing Technique*…allow your breathing to be produced by your structure and movement…be breathed by the motion of your movement and structure…*Control Pause*…Performance Breathing Exercise…balances health and performance…through practice exceeds the gains of Power Breathing

The best way to learn a new skill… *Elementary Motor Component*… *Biomechanical Exercise™*…Kinetic Chain…Forward Engineering…*Reverse Engineering*…*Lateral Engineering*…*movement-in-between*…There is only transition

r

INTRODUCTION

By Steven Barnes

About forty years ago a bully followed me home from Alta Loma Elementary School. I was eight, and he punched me in the stomach all the way home. Every time I tried to cover my stomach, he threatened to punch me in the face.

I'd pretty much buried that memory until the age of forty, until a self-hypnosis session discovered that buried memory, burrowed into my subconscious, had driven a lifetime of extreme fear response to sparring class, as a result slowed my progress in the arts and associated far too much distress with the experience. That beating had anchored together with a lifetime of other humiliations to create the psychological equivalent of the Gordian Knot.

For thirty years I went from teacher to teacher, asking if any could help heal the emotional response that deviled me. Although many were wonderful teachers of physical skills, none of them had a practical answer in this less tangible aspect of the Way. So thrown on my own resources I assembled a patchwork of self-improvement techniques: Psycho-Cybernetics, NLP, self-hypnosis, contemporary shamanism, Ericksonian hypnosis, several styles of meditation, several styles of yoga, therapy and more to enable me to keep "moving forward." And all I ever wanted was what I'd never had: sheer joy in motion.

Along the way, I earned *dan* rankings in Judo and Karate, and spent years as Kung Fu Columnist for _Black Belt_ magazine, so although the emotional issues remained, I couldn't say that I wasn't having a good time.

One day, about two years ago a former training partner named Dr. Eric Cobb e-mailed me and mentioned a man named Scott Sonnon, describing his physical attributes in, what seemed to me, rather fantastical terms. *Well, all right*, I thought. *Let's see what he's got.* I purchased a couple of his tapes, and was especially impressed by _Be Breathed_ and its concept of *Perpetual Exercise*. Next up was the _Flow State Performance Spiral_ audio tape stayed in my car stereo for a month, and I listened to it around twenty times.

I was blown away by Coach Sonnon's intelligence, real-world knowledge, and creativity. And his quality of motion was, I thought, remarkable. As an action-adventure novelist for twenty-five years I'd *written* about people who moved like water over rocks, but never actually *seen* one.

Taking a chance, I dropped a note to Scott. Despite the fact that he was on vacation with his family, he was kind enough to write a multi-page reply, offering his insights on the effects of fear-reactivity on the human body and mind. His generosity blew me away. I decided to attend the first Clubbell certification workshop as a way of meeting Scott, and despite a moderate case of butterflies, went off to Seattle.

I found Coach Sonnon and his crew to be great folks, generous and approachable. Scott himself was even more skilled than he had appeared on his tapes, with a wacky sense of humor. Smart funny people impress me. Those who can counter anything I can throw without having to get out of low gear impress me even more.

But the workshop was about more than learning how to swing Clubbells. To my surprise, Clubbells were just the outer expression of a body-mind disciple Coach Sonnon called *Maximology*. I'd heard of *Zdorovye*, the Russian health system, but what was *this*..? It seemed that in just the few short months I'd been observing, this stuff was evolving right in front of my eyes. In *Zdorovye*, there was much useful discussion of breathing, motion and alignment, but in *Maximology* he had synthesized a vast number of wrestling, gymnastic and general movement drills into something even more formidable. We barely touched a Clubbell that first day, spending most of our time in core-agility exercises. It was my first contact with what Scott calls *Biomechanical Exercise*™, and I call magic.

After Sunday, I felt like I'd gotten five times my money's worth, but a couple of days later something more remarkable happened. I was driving down the street, and my mind started free-associating, and it went back to that forty-year old painful memory of being punched in the stomach…*and I couldn't access it*. I almost swerved off the street. Over the next days I tried to pull that memory up, and couldn't. Every time I tried to, every time I visualized that bully hitting me in the stomach, I watched my mental self use my thirty odd years of training to dump him on his ass. What was this? I hadn't been working on those issues lately…

I talked with Coach Sonnon about it, and he explained that high-level neural repatterning sometimes causes such core change. I couldn't believe it. Over thirty years of grief, years of therapy and work, and ninety-percent of the problem were gone in *two days*?

And that hadn't even been the point of the exercise? I was hooked.

Coach Sonnon is a phenomenal source of over-all knowledge of combative mental and physical conditioning, and a walking advertisement for said knowing.

In the pages that follow, Coach Sonnon mentions the acronym **F.E.A.R.** (**F**alse **E**vidence **A**ppearing **R**eal). It also means **F**%$# **E**verything **A**nd **R**un. Nothing stops our excellence, dooms us to mediocrity and lost dreams, like our own fear. No one can stop us like us. Whether in career, love, or health, our sense of limitations creates chaos in our lives where there should be power and grace. And what is worse, once a pattern is engrained, we can become *afraid of being afraid*, in a mirror-maze of self-depreciation and self-examination that is difficult to escape.

The answer is the body. Your body remembers, deep in its cells, the dance of health, the "original configuration" of your human hardware/software bundle, before you loaded in all the buggy, conflicting, cobble-together social programs, each authority figure or frame of reference or intense "learning experience" competing to tell you who and what you are.

Proper use of your body hits the "reset" button. If the student is willing it is possible to move the body to reach the spirit: masters have known this for centuries. I believe that Coach Sonnon has found an almost uniquely powerful and direct tool to personal mastery. This is the book I wish I could have read decades ago, the very book.

I envy you so: I had to wait forty years for _Body-Flow_. You only have to wait until you turn the page.

--April 16, 2003
Steven Barnes
Longview, Washington

WHAT IS BODY-FLOW?

"I am skeptical of science's presumption of objectivity and definitiveness. I have a difficult time seeing scientific results, especially in neurobiology, as anything but provisional approximations, to be enjoyed for a while and discarded as soon as better accounts become available." - Antonio Damasio, Descartes' Error

In his prologue to this book, Ken Harper describes *Body-Flow* as the ability to be "fully present in the moment," a state of unity in which the mind, body and spirit act together. As I will explain in this book, *Body-Flow* holds the key to better health and well being through this integrated presence.

Many people discus how to gain flow in life, but the very investigation taints the exploration. They ask, "How do I gain *Body-Flow*?" However, it is this very inquiry that arrests the development of 95% of those who seek physical and mental improvement.

Body-Flow is *not* something to be *gained*. *This* is the reason most people do not know how to flow. *Body-Flow* is not something you do, but something which you must get out of the way of. You must get out of the way of your own genius, talent and abundance – which are your birthright. *Body-Flow* is not something to be acquired, but rather something that you will learn to avoid interrupting.

A much more appropriate question to ask is: what prevents you from having *Body-Flow*?

Many people perceive flow as the absence of errors, the condition of never experiencing surprise and shock; never fearing challenge. This is why they are not masterful; why they lack grace and poise. They associate "doing their best" with perfection. This creates fear of making mistakes by creating false expectations of performance.

But it is precisely the experience of failure which opens the gateway to flow. The failures are just scenery. Winston Churchill said, *"Success is going from failure to failure without losing enthusiasm."* Successful people systematically unhinge themselves from failed expectations. They move from one attachment to the next without being distracted by the appearance of failure. Flow isn't something you seek, but rather it is the process you unlock by letting go of attachments, by freeing yourself from expectations.

Dance annotator Rudolph Laban coined the term *Bound-Flow*, the stopping point in action. So we can define success as the enthusiastic movement from failure to failure without attachment or expectation - without binding-flow.

Ask yourself, "What is my current degree of success?" How long does it take you to recover from being surprised, shocked, disappointed, frustrated, angered, dismayed, or any other emotional or mental distraction? How quickly can you regain your composure, your enthusiasm and stop resisting the flow of life?

You must challenge or change the training habits and personal beliefs that contribute to your stress and dysfunction – to the blockage of your flow. What is it that you put in your own way? What hurdles do you create for yourself?

Masterful people perceive making mistakes as a positive influence on performance. They perceive the unexpected as opportunity meeting preparation.

The key to **Body-Flow**, therefore, rests with deliberate exposure to making mistakes and to unexpected events, combined with the proper training protocol, emotional control and mental attitude. **Body-Flow** systematically removes fear of making mistakes and fear of the unexpected. Your ability to take risks allows you to enter greatness and uncover your personal mastery.

Face challenge by risking mistakes and welcoming unexpected events. Deliberately engage in the areas which you fear. You increase your confidence not by refinement in areas in which you are comfortable, but by facing the areas in which you fear mistakes and the unknown. Your fears inhibit your performance and block your flow.

Flow never *attaches* anywhere. It never *abides*. It constantly moves. You must focus on this state of *detachment* in order for you to address constantly changing variables.

Seek your freedom. Keep your movement from binding. In reality, stillness can be gained only through continual motion, since attempting to stop motion requires force. You always move, even when you try to force yourself to be still.

WHAT ARE THE DANGERS OF BOUND-FLOW?

When your flow is bound, it's like walking across a mud-lined river. Your feet sink and you become mired to your knees in the muck. Each step requires every ounce of effort you can muster and all the while, people, opportunities and life itself seems to be floating by...

Think of *Bound-Flow* as a pattern of knots in your muscles, making it difficult to breath, stand and sit straight, painful to move. It's difficult, painful, and energetically expensive to move with these networks of muscular tethers, isn't it? You bet it is!

When addressing *Bound-Flow*, analysis begets paralysis. You can't think your way out of a cage, especially if the cage is self-imposed and despite the fact that the bars are invisible. As you'll discover throughout **Body-Flow**, no amount of pop psychology will DO anything about your movement. You need to ACT, to MOVE in order to cast off the shackles to your health, strength and performance.

To free yourself from the bondage of *Bound-Flow*, you need to make the invisible bars of the cage visible. You need to identify what keeps you in, and by doing so, secure your path to liberate your health, to secure pain-free movement, and to tap into your literally unlimited potential.

The first thing you must do is realize that coordination, grace, poise, agility, balance... these attributes are not learned. They are your birthright, your genetic inheritance. What you learn, what you condition and make repeatable are the opposite.

The second step in your emancipation from mediocrity involves understanding how you came to systematically build two types of restraints to your flow. By learning how you built this cage, you can deconstruct it and simply... walk away from unhealthy, weak, poor performance lifestyle patterns.

WHERE ARE THE BARS TO THE CAGE?

There are two types of bars to your cage, two degrees of *Bound-Flow*: the kind where you **forget how** to flow and the kind where you **resist** flow.

The first manner of bars is where you just have forgotten your ability to flow. **Sensory Motor Amnesia** (SMA) is a phrase coined by renowned therapist Thomas Hanna. *"This is a condition,"* he said, *"in which the sensory-motor neurons of the voluntary cortex have lost some portion of their ability to control all or some of the muscles of the body. Sensory motor amnesia occurs neither as an organic lesion of the brain nor of the musculoskeletal system; it occurs as a functional deficit whereby the ability to contract a muscle group has been surrendered to sub-cortical reflexes. These reflexes will chronically contract muscles at a programmed rate – ten percent, thirty percent, sixty percent, or whatever – and the voluntary cortex is powerless to relax these muscles below that programmed rate. It has lost and forgotten the ability to do so."*

In essence, SMA is a 'forgotten' and 'ignored' habitual pattern of muscular contraction somewhere in the body. This loss has a tremendous impact on all aspects of our health, strength, fitness and performance.

For most people, this will make no "sense" until you can sense what you have lost. Basically, you don't miss what you can't remember. As we will see, there is hope. There are tools, methods, processes and programs to **Body-Flow** that will help dust off the cobwebs on your natural grace, poise and energy.

But there is another danger created by *Bound-Flow*: where you **resist** the natural course of events. This resistance is due to tension being stored in the muscles when not needed for activity. Called **Residual Muscle Tension** this is closely related to SMA. RMT often relates to the presence of an unconsciously held partial contraction of muscles following prolonged periods of stress or activity. While not as habitual as SMA, residual muscle tension is the bane of every person's physical freedom and every athlete's performance and strength. RMT interferes with rest, recovery, and relaxation by disintegrating proper performance-related neurological coordination and function. It aches, limits movement capability and eventually leads to SMA.

RMT can create SMA through *Avoidance Syndrome*. If it hurts to move in a certain way, then you consciously or unconsciously tend to avert from the pain. However, like any form of conditioning, the more you do something, the more you make that activity repeatable. And once you make that activity repeatable, you "progress."

I introduced this in my book *Clubbell Training for Circular Strength* (RMAX.tv Productions, 2002) named the *"Laws of Conditioning:"* every action is an act of conditioning:

<u>Law of Outcome</u>: Whatever you do produces an outcome, regardless of how you value that outcome.

<u>Law of Adaptation</u>: Whatever you do over a period of time creates a change in you to find homeostasis, regardless of how you value that adaptation.

<u>Law of Progress</u>:   Whatever you do with continually increasing volume, intensity, density, or complexity becomes more easily repeatable, regardless of how you value the progress.

Progression refers to the body's adaptation to a certain repeated behavior. For instance, if you experience daily emotional stress such as verbal abuse and/or consistent physical abuse, you may tend to lift the shoulders and transpose the neck forward with the face downward facing. The more that this occurs, the more the body adapts... by building muscle tissue and reinforcing the sustained tension in the neck, shoulders and back. Make no mistake about this – it IS muscle-building; muscle that is rock-hard, highly irritable, and very inflexible with limited range of motion. This "Defensive Bracing" impacts the musculature, which in turn impacts the structural alignment of the skeleton, which leads to a host of dangerous internal conditions.

The following chart, *Wheel of Dis-Ease*, I created to use when I teach health care professionals to help them better address the TRUE needs of their patients. This book, for the sake of brevity and for streamlining it to help your performance, strength and health, and unlock your natural talent, genius and abundance need not get highly technical.

Wheel of Dis-Ease

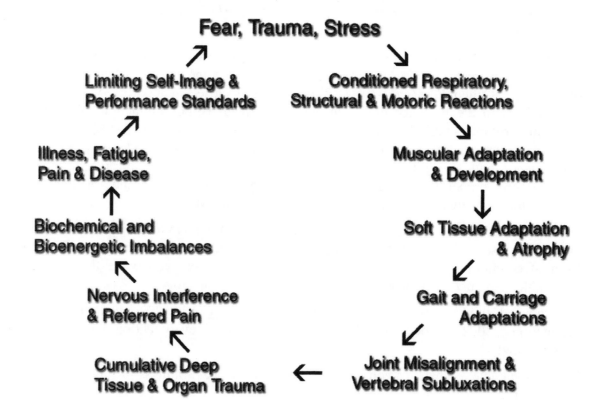

Sensory Motor Amnesia and *Residual Muscular Tension* directly impact your movement capabilities and as a result contribute to binding your flow. As you can see from the *Wheel of Dis-Ease*, SMA and RMT contribute to a vicious perpetuating cycle – a downward spiraling feedback loop of diminishing health, strength and performance.

However, the direct impact isn't the greatest threat to your health, strength and performance as I've alluded to above. The most significant hazard to your well being regards how these two, SMA and RMT, directly impact your self-image, self-confidence and self-determination (perceived autonomy) and lead to illness, disease and chronic conditions.

WHAT IS FEAR-REACTIVITY?

Again and again, people ask me, *"What is **Fear-Reactivity**? Where are my natural talent, genius and abundance?"* Every time I respond that your natural talent, genius and abundance lay underneath **Fear-Reactivity**.

Fear-Reactivity is the non-specific, conditioned pattern of concrete, observable behavior involving movement, breathing and structural alignment; as opposed to the internal event such as catastrophic thinking or emotional anxiety or panic.

At the time of writing this, I am overcoming a coffee addiction – one of the few drawbacks to living in the Pacific Northwest of the United States of America is coffee so powerful one cup could power a small city.

This morning, as I always do, I grabbed my fan mail to head up on the Mountain to practice and then cool down by reading the letters from my friends and clients.

Today was another unique epiphany in that it was one or two days away from concluding a restoration period after walking one step too far into Over-Training. Pushing the envelope; increasing the threshold of pain to increase the threshold of performance, often means hovering on the brink of injury, in order to stimulate the organism to adapt and progress. However, progress is often the villain. Your progress can conceal your **Body-Flow**, if you misinterpret **Body-Flow** as compilation and not distillation of performance, health and strength.

The run up the Mountain is not one lacking challenge. Most athletes go into significant aerobic debt just walking up its steep grade. However, I do this daily and for years and for me… the challenge is inside, not conquering the Mountain. Nature always wins, because she's a Mother. But she's not our opponent, is she? She's a vehicle to challenge ourselves, to leverage out our ego and find the essence of who we are, by burning away who we are not.

And there you have it. It is the burning away of that which is not us. What melts off as slag metal is **Fear-Reactivity**. In the cauldron of practice, training and competition we assault that personality doppelganger which with raucous antics parades around in our heads. This ego can take us on a lifetime stumbling from one tangent to the next, a seductive roller coaster which abuses us with "entertainment" as well as malice.

So, I burn up the Mountain, observing my breathing, finding my gait's groove, sending my mind to the day's new pattern of tensions. But this day, as I ran, my mind became pre-occupied with the core elements of my philosophy – Synergy, Flow and Harmony. As I meditated on those precepts, I become "lost" or rather I "lost time" with the exertion of my daily Journey.

I'm sure you've all done this. Lost time. Gone on autopilot. Hit the Zone. My life has been a seemingly endless pursuit for that Zone, as many of the people who have been with me for these decades of physical culture know all too well. I've lost friends and family because of addictions, including to my addiction to optimal human performance in fighting and martial arts.

But it was only today, as I dedicated myself to composing the ideal method of crafting this description of *Fear-Reactivity* did I totally realize it myself. All my life culminated in this one thing, this one realization, which it seems I've struggled and strained and stressed to discover.

I am not my addictions.

YOU are not YOUR addictions.

Think of it this way. Your body becomes aroused to threats in a specific method. When you receive some sort of stimulus, you have a specific, learned and conditioned pattern of muscular tension, structural alignment and respiratory behavior which is unique to you. That tension, position and breathing elicits a hormonal release, sometime slow, sometimes a dump. Each of those chemical brews creates an emotional feeling within you, and each of those feelings is anchored with the family of similar experiences. So when you experience the feeling of one of these you have mental impressions, frames of reference if you will, to similar events. Those impressions give rise to internal dialogue, evaluation of the experience, judgments… "thoughts."

You go through that process a million times a day in a fraction of a second, instantly collecting data, processing and internally representing, then interacting with your environment.

Today, as I ran to the summit of the Mountain, I experienced something euphoric. My feet began to barely pad the surface of the ground. I felt near floating, my respiration as normal as if I were sitting at my desk typing, and my alignment as if I were being hung from a marionette string – crown to coccyx. Exhilarating. Spectacular. Truly awe-some.

I thanked the Heaven's for the experience, nearly gloating at the gift. Today I felt free from the anguished withdrawal symptoms of recovering from a coffee addiction. For me that's no small event. I have by nature a highly addictive personality. I've had to overcome addictions to nearly all of civilization's so-called "blessings" – nicotine, alcohol, sugar, as well as life's pleasures such as addictions to sex, adoration, fame, wealth, conquest/fighting and even exercise. Addiction is easy for someone who is very passionate.

Coffee had snuck up on me because of my lack of vigilance, with some arrogance mixed in to the pot. I had chosen to vanquish the foe because my heart began to pump just a wee bit uncomfortably too resounding during my training. No major problem now, but my gut told me that in 10 years, I would have to deal with some serious heart problems if I didn't cut off this medusa's head now. So fell another opponent. But like any good (bad) action movie, I left the room before the enemy perished, and he snuck up and bit me in the can.

The experience of running up the Mountain today was a product of pushing through the withdrawal symptoms. Biochemically, I forced myself through a barrier and my neurological system faced with distress of withdrawal AND physical exertion, adapted. It dumped a tremendous wash of wonderful chemicals into my system, such as epinephrine (adrenaline) and endorphins (morphine basically). What a High! What a fabulous fix!

Wait a minute! Fix. High. Wait just a damn minute! That sounds incredibly like a dysfunctional pattern of behavior with which I'm all too acquainted… addiction.

Half way through my practice, I realized that I had ceased meditating on my breathing through my exercises. But simultaneous to returning into my body, I realized that the euphoria was in the midst of being replaced. Replaced with my old childhood arch nemesis – hypoglycemia (HG).

HG was not such a big threat to me when I was a punk kid, because I would just kick him out the door by pounding down the white flour, processed sugars, caffeine, and any other stimulant I could find. Crash you say? Never! I had more Snacky-snacks with which to fill the seats of my digestive roller coaster.

But since my nutritional revolution a few years ago, off the stimulants, off the junk, and only real, organic, free-range whole foods (though still recovering from "organic coffee"), I've come to battle HG with religious fervor. Constantly throughout the day, but seemingly now on a regular schedule, he comes strolling in the door. When he does, I'm usually busy, writing, training, playing with my family, even sometimes he comes and kicks me in the can while I'm in the midst of preparing food, because I neglected to get the meal in my gullet 20 minutes before he was due to arrive at my house.

In the midst of my practice on the Mountain, he hit me. He hit me like he's damn never hit me before and I almost buckled at the knees. I knew it was a danger to remain for too long up on the Mountain like that, so I pondered heading back down before having even sat down to read my mail. Damn it, I exclaimed to myself. Stupid. I mismanaged myself again. I neglected to forecast the frequency and intensity of today's peak and valley.

Funny that I thought to myself – Peak and Valley. Up to the top for the euphoria, back down to the valley's bottom for dealing with the stress. Funny how that has been literal for me my entire life.

I've always scrambled up the Mountain. All my life struggling for that Peak Experience, for the Optimal Performance, for the Zone. All my life I've detested the boredom, the mundaneness of average existence and its lack-luster dullness, the gray, the blah.

Today I tried to ease up on criticizing myself. It was an oath I pledged to my family because that criticism has started to ooze into my behavior with them. I started to impose my perfectionism, my idealism, my dreaded addiction to the Peak, upon them and their occasional inadequacies. I realized that if I were to show more compassion for my family, I needed to start with my own internal dialogue. Admittedly though this was not my original thought. My family prodded me to do this because they realized how precariously I was balanced upon the pedestal I had mounted.

So, I backed off the judgmental attack on my poor timing of my Peak and Valley – of letting HG kick my ass again. I said to myself, "this is not you speaking. You are not your frustration, anger, lack of energy and disappointment. It is just a chemical attack of HG, no more no less real than a phantom."

But that's when it hit me. How could the Valley be an illusion and not the Peak? How could I tell myself that I am not the Valley, if I am saying all these years, through all these experiences, through this 20 odd year pursuit of Peak Experience?

I could not. I had to accept that I was neither Peak nor Valley. If the chemical experience of HG's assault upon my senses amounted to no more than biochemical warfare producing a range of feelings, impressions and dialogue… then I had to accept that the adaptation of my organism to overcoming the resistance of unique stressors was equally not ME!

I am not my addiction to the Peak.

You see, the organism cycles through this process each time it is exposed to stimuli:

Stimulus: any novel or noxious event.

<u>Sensations</u>: your collection of information through your senses and transmission of that signal through to the Central Nervous System.

<u>Autonomic arousal</u>: heart rate, respiration, blood pressure, internal temperature, blood flow shift, etc.

<u>Hormonal arousal</u>: release or dump of various chemicals into the system to super-charge the system to fight or flee.

<u>Feelings</u>: each pattern of tension, breathing, structure, and chemical blend becomes a particular feeling; one is happiness, one sadness; one is frustration, one exhilaration; one is anger, one lust.

<u>Impressions</u>: each feeling is categorized by similar experiences. When you have one feeling, it is anchored to similar experiences. You judge an event by the feeling you have, and those judgments categorize your experiences.

<u>Thoughts</u>: as you make instant judgments, you react by creating inner discussion regarding your impression of what you have just experienced. Some thoughts are negative, some positive, each of course dependent upon this process.

This is a very general, very elementary explanation of the process. It's highly sophisticated. More sophisticated than nearly all but a very few experts in psychophysiology, neurobiology, stress physiology and behavioral science comprehend. But you get the gist.

The conclusions that we draw here are monumental! Feelings come before (create) thoughts is the first that come to mind! But that's only the first half. The second half of that statement is your muscle tension, movement, structural alignment and breathing come before (create) your feelings. Ever hear the saying, *"if you want happiness, then smile?"*

But that's not the most impacting, most humbling, most numbing admission.

If a dangerous stimulus elicits this process, producing a response, and if that stimulus-response is conditioned, and if you adapt and progress upon that conditioning, who are you that is not a mere reaction to that stimulus? Who are you that is not that addictive compulsion to knee-jerk events in your life? Who is this doppelganger that lives your life in your place?

If you are not that reflex, not that pattern of tension, not those dumped chemicals, not those phantom pains and feelings, not those impressions and not that dialogue, and not those knee-jerk reactions to those stressors, who... are... you?

Who you are, what you are capable of achieving lay beneath that process. Who you truly are, your natural abundance, talent and genius lay concealed by that conditioned *Fear-Reactivity*. Who you are is what is left when you burn away the slag which is your fears.

Who you are is the slab of marble. Remove everything that is not your greatness. What remains is your *Body-Flow*.

Fear-Reactivity is a term I coined referring to a learned, conditioned reaction to stress, shock or trauma. It embeds in each of us; no one escapes it. And in the modern world, we are beset with stressors like no other time in history. Worse still is that we biologically cannot differentiate between an emotional/symbolic threat and an actual physical threat. If a boss or co-worker is belligerent in our face screaming at us, we become aroused (without proper training) in the same way that we would if someone held a knife to our throat.

We haven't evolved to accommodate our new post-modernistic lifestyle. We're Stone Age bodies living in a digital world. Our physiology differs not at all from when we chased down Woolly Mammoths and gathered berries. We still have the potential to track game and gather food, but we don't have a way to release all that stress, and we don't have a way to distinguish between true threats and false threats. Or as the anonymous acronym states, distinguish between evidence and F.E.A.R. – *False Evidence Appearing Real*.

TOLERANCE TO STRESS: ADAPTATION AND PROGRESS OF FEAR-REACTIVITY

As you'll read, the true villain is the nature in which we learn. Any activity which is sustained, we adapt to. We become more tolerant of that level of activity. This includes stress, shock and trauma – which account for debilitating conditions such as ***Post-Traumatic Stress Disorder*** (PTSD) is traumatic stress which has not been relieved through a working through of trauma and is of sufficient severity to decrease a person's ability to function in life.

But the hazard to our lives comes from this ability of our organism to adapt to any situation. We can adapt to over-eating or under-eating, lethargy or liveliness, Peak or Valley. The more we do something, the more we adapt to make that repeatable. The good thing about this is that we progress in strength, health, fitness, happiness, and performance. The bad thing about this is that we progress in weakness, disease, fatness, unhappiness and poor performance. The most important thing to remember is that they are all outcomes. We choose to attach negative and positive associations to these.

However, at any time we can change them, by beginning anew, by breaking the pattern and altering our behavior. Baby steps. As stated by the institutional credo of my Strength Magazine, named *Full Circle* (www.circularstrengthmag.com), *"A New Beginning Determines the End."*

But before we go in to how to interrupt patterns and reframe them positively, we must see the most detrimental impact ***Fear-Reactivity*** has on us.

At any point in your life, there are events and situations which cause within you differing intensity and duration of stress; consider it a continuum from low to medium to high stress, depicted in the ***Stress Arousal Scale***.

<u>Stress Arousal Scale</u>

<u>Hypo-Arousal</u>: low activation of your *Parasympathetic Nervous System* (PNS). Your breathing is easy, deep; and your pulse – slow; your skin tone – normal.

<u>Low Arousal</u>: low to moderate PNS activation combined with low activation of the *Sympathetic Nervous System* (SNS). Your breathing and pulse increase though your skin color remains normal; OR your skin may become pale and glisten without increasing your breathing and pulse.

<u>Moderate Arousal</u>: increased SNS arousal. Your skin becomes pale. Your heart rate and breathing rapid.

<u>High Arousal</u>: dramatic increases in SNS arousal. Your heart rate accelerates, as does your respiration. Your skin becomes very pale and you get the cold sweats.

<u>Hyper-Arousal</u>: dramatic increases in SNS and PNS. Though your skin stays pale, your heart rate drops off very low; OR your pupils dilate and your face flushes with color; OR your heart rate drops and your breathing gets shallow and rapid; OR your breathing becomes very slow but your heart rate races.

However, like all things, the longer you sustain an activity, the more you adapt and progress to make that activity repeatable. In the case of stress, you become more tolerant. So in reference to the Stress Arousal Scale, your base level doesn't return to No Arousal. You stay at Low Arousal all the time. Smaller and smaller things seem to "set you off." And this is just the first stage. You grow even more tolerant, and Moderate Arousal becomes your "normal" state. You're in some serious trouble at that point!

Like becoming tolerant to a drug, you can take higher dosages to get the original effect – that's the nature of addiction. In the case of stress, as you become more tolerant, you accept more stress than before, but come to accept that as the norm, as average. Many people live with dangerous levels of stress, daily, because they've come to accept it as normal. Many people live with abuse (and self-abuse) because they adapted and progressed, becoming tolerant of their terrible situations.

HOW DOES TOLERANCE IMPACT MY HEALTH, STRENGTH AND PERFORMANCE?

Fear-Reactivity is your nervous system's conditioned reaction to perceived dangers, pain and trauma. You have likely heard the term referred to as "shock" in cases of physical harm or accidents. That is its most extreme occurrence. *Fear-Reactivity* also occurs under lesser forms of threat, and even when the body is not actually harmed, such as when you step down expecting another stair when there is none, when you think something flies at your head when it was only a shadow, or when you think that you left your wallet or business document at home and come to find it only a moment later.

Prey may create *Fear-Reactivity* when stalked by predators whether or not they are caught and eaten. In the case of modern life, this can take the shape of feeling that someone follows you, of anticipating an angered spouse or belligerent employer's wrath, or embarrassment of public speaking.

Very simply, in threat - the typical escape reaction is to *fight, flight or freeze*. The reaction is assisted by the Sympathetic branch of the Autonomic Nervous System: blood flow comes strongly to the muscles of the limbs, breathing increases, heart rate increases, blood pressure increases, internal temperature increases, digestion and waste elimination are inhibited (or instantly evacuated to assist *fight or flight*); the system is in all-alert, condition red.

After the event is over, the nervous system releases an alarm inhibitor (cortisol) and it will usually return these body systems to a normal level of functioning within a few hours, days or weeks (depending upon intensity, duration, frequency or complexity of the stressors).

Sometimes we are unable to make sense of the threatening event – if it's too intense, lasts too long, happens too frequently, or is too complex. Our nervous system doesn't get the message that the traumatic event is over and that we have survived. The chemical signal is insufficient to halt the alarm reactions and we become more and more aroused. We get caught in a feedback loop continuing to signal the nervous system to prepare the body. The result is we freeze in place… paralyzed.

The continued preparation for defensive action is at the core of the disturbing physical and psychological symptoms associated with traumatic stress. It disturbs your sleep, makes your concentration difficult, leads to panic attacks, extreme startle reflex, rapid or irregular heartbeat, cold sweats, hyper-activity, exhaustion and fatigue. Psychological symptoms include: anxiety, feeling unsafe, flashbacks, nightmares, avoidance of situations, thoughts and feelings that carry reminders of the traumatic event, feeling detached from oneself or others.

If a threat is repeated before you have had time to recover, or if you perceive yourself as caught, the Parasympathetic branch will also come into play and may even "mask" the Sympathetic, i.e.: blood may flow to the center of the body, respiration decrease, and heart rate drop, while the skin becomes cold, and paralysis, or *Tonic Immobility* will occur.

Tonic Immobility is loosely defined as a state of prolonged muscular contraction. Ironically that is the same definition for being "muscle-bound." *Tonic Immobility* is a state of profound motor inhibition typically elicited by a high-fear situation. Specific features include a temporary paralysis, tremors/shaking, inability to call out or scream, loss of consciousness/feinting, numbness and insensitivity to pain, sensation of feeling cold.

From feinting goats dropping over from loud noise to paralyzing silky sharks by grabbing their tail, the antelope that suddenly stops struggling while in the lions jaws, the deer frozen in headlights; all exemplify *tonic immobility*.

The most severe cases of this is **Post-Traumatic Stress**, which can result from any traumatic situation in which a person's life is at risk or where s/he perceives it as such. Examples include: war, surgery, rape, sudden loss, assault, abuse, and accidents. **Fear-Reactivity** can begin from individual events such as an accident. Or they can be linked in chains: abuse, torture (which usually involves several incidents over time). When this trauma and fear are not worked through at the time of occurrence -- usually because adequate help, support, safety and contact was not available -- psychological and physical symptoms can develop. Typical complaints include: phobias, panic attacks, night terrors, dizziness and fainting, heart palpitations, tremors, feeling paralyzed to act, speak, decide when under stress, and other "unexplainable" physical symptoms.

Sound pretty awful? Well, <u>everyone</u> who faces stress of any sort suffers this, differing only in degree! If you harbor fears, have been called defensive, feel that you could be embarrassed, are volatile, can be easily angered or aroused, irritable, have anxieties, fears or trepidations, or the whole host of non-fun living, then you are subject to the above.

Remember, we become tolerant – we produce outcomes, adapt, and progress. We embed **Fear-Reactivity** and it becomes the norm.

It is **Fear-Reactivity** which must be removed. Natural synergy, harmony and flow lay underneath the armor which you've created. You don't need that rusty suit of plate mail. Take it off and cast it away!

Fear-Reactivity is what binds your flow. To get out of the way of your natural, abundant **Body-Flow**, you need to do one thing – diminish and eliminate **Fear-Reactivity**.

BOUND-FLOW AND SELF-IMAGE

I know you may think, "OF COURSE! These are fabulous discoveries and explanations! But I still have to get up in the morning, get my family prepared for the day, change diapers, deal with co-workers, et cetera. How do I remove *Fear-Reactivity* in reality?!"

Great question. I'll give you the answer. Remember that *Body-Flow* is not a compilation of skills, but rather the **diminishing, the recovery from and eventual elimination of Bound-Flow**. To uncover and amplify your natural energy, poise and grace, you need to remove *Fear-Reactivity*… daily!

So now you have to actually implement this, right? But it's not as oppressive and ominous as you may first think. Definitely, this will take daily practice. Each day you need to apply it against the resistance that life creates for us – or rather that we manifest for ourselves to evolve. This is what I call Natural Competition. It is facing resistance and overcoming the lull of lethargy, the seduction to wane in your dedication to Deepening your Daily Practice.

You can do it. It can be done. Many have done it. And all successful people do it. It is not complicated, though it will become sophisticated, because you will weave this into every fiber of your existence… to ferret out where *Fear-Reactivity* resides, where *Bound-Flow* occurs.

So, let's look at the process. You constantly deal with stress, right? If you're an animate creature you do. Even a rock endures stress. But we'd all prefer not being the rock wouldn't we? We'd all like to be the river.

Basically the process goes like this: if you react in the same way, over mobilized, adrenalined, pissing vinegar and flaming on, you reinforce that behavioral pattern. When you feel this way, your muscles get tense, right? Everyone's muscles get coiled and rock-hard if they allow the stress to get to them. And if it's a novel, sudden, frequent, or intense level of stress, everyone must RECOVER FROM that sudden knotting of muscle, that "muscle-bound" feeling that stress elicits.

In my long history as a fighter and a fight coach, this was my most significant work – the recovery process from shock, surprise, from perceived failure and from overwhelmed or over-aggressive behavior. We fighters are such simple-minded folk. We become so highly focused, so singular in our concentration that we often end up with a face full of bark, never seeing that proverbial forest through the trees. We fixate on skill acquisition and refinement – looking to get that perfect takedown, that sweet box, that fresh submission. As a result, fighters, only after their careers are long over, realize what their coaches attempted to advise them – the key is not about the daily increase, but rather the daily decrease.

It's not about acquiring advanced skills, not about gaining perfection. As I wrote in the beginning *Body-Flow* is not something you pursue. *Body-Flow* is something that you get out of the way of. *Bound-Flow* is what inhibits performance, strength and health. Muscle-boundedness hemorrhages performance – it "leaks" efficiency and it "drains" your effectiveness.

So the goal when it came to fighting, any form, and any sport, regards RECOVERING from that binding, from perceived failure and from shock and surprise WHEN it happens. Mistakes are a guarantee, like death and taxes. But the truly great, the successful, talented and abundant, all share one common trait: <u>they all recover quickly from mistakes</u>. They each **unbind** more rapidly than others. They avoid falling into the feedback loop of frustration. They do not try to stop their mistakes by becoming more tense. They realize that <u>tension is a CHOICE</u>!

An arrogant fighter takes an extremely long time to recover from perceived failures, from shock, and from surprise. His Pattern competes for his ability to perceive and respond to the actual events as they occur. His ego gets in the way of his performance, slowing him down, decreasing his discernment, increasing the gap between the mistake and his ability to get back in the saddle.

An anxious fighter tends to rapidly fall into a cycle, becomes easily entrapped by a Pattern – the doubts, hesitations, the insecurities he wears on his gloves. They're simple to observe. Just like the arrogant fighter, the anxious fighter intervenes on his ability to ACT – to respond to the situation. He becomes paralyzed by his own fears, prey to his own doubts, and forgets how to recover.

Now the field of battle is no different than the field of business, no different than the field of sport, no different than the field of life, in general. How could it be? Life interweaves. Fighting however is the *micro of the macro*, and it allowed me some special opportunities to realize some unique insights. If you haven't figured it out by now, if you DON'T "get" these insights if you're a fighter, then you become a human punching bag for the rest of your life. You really have no option in martial arts. You either get "it" or you get "feedback" until you do.

But this is where martial arts transfer into everyday experience. It's what the "Greats" truly understand. Don't interchange "Greats" with 'masters.' A 'master' (or "expert" or whatever vogue title) is a rank given to those who can demonstrate a curriculum of skills. A 'Great' is someone who can adapt his or her knowledge into every new venue encountered. (And a 'coach' is someone who can "lift-up" others to realize their inherent greatness.)

You experience this every day, in every moment. The goal is to recognize *Bound-Flow* as it occurs, and recover from it quickly – rather than facilitating it and getting stuck in a feedback loop of increasing tension. If you do this, if you increase your awareness of binding, then you begin to gain options. You can't do anything if you're not aware of the problem, so awareness is the first step.

Later, I'll be drafting you a map, so that you may plot your own unique course to uncovering your **Body-Flow** – your genius, talent and abundance.

So how does Fear-Reactivity specifically surface in me?

Tension

Well, think of it this way, when you're angry, you condition your muscles to tense in a certain way, from clenching your jaw to wrinkling your forehead to arching your head forwards aggressively. If you are intimidated or overwhelmed, crawling in on yourself, caving in, submitting, fleeing from confrontation, accepting abuse, guess what? You reinforce that behavioral pattern as well. You condition your muscles to tense in a certain way from lifting your shoulders, wincing your eyes, looking down at the ground, crossing your arms, hunching your back, shuffling your feet.

Breath

Not only your muscular tension and skeletal position are affected, but your breathing as well. You breathe rapidly, shallow, gasping, holding your breath. Your blood courses through you as your heart pumps hard and fast… fluttering occasionally, pounding (no referent) Each pattern of movement, structural alignment and breathing manufactures that hormonal dump into your system, supercharging your body with no release, no cathartic emission to discharge that toxic chemical brew from your system. You become your own biohazard, and you reinforce it each time you react to the same fear with the same patterned reaction.

Think about it. If certain things stress you out, and those sensations cause an autonomic arousal (muscle tension, heart rate, blood pressure, breathing pattern, et cetera), it directly creates the hormonal arousal (dumping all those chemicals into your system), and that hormonal arousal influences your emotional feelings. Those feelings anchor to impressions and those impressions erupt as thoughts.

Reactivity

It happens thousands of times a day. The question is – **do you deliberately choose your response, or are you a product of reactions?** The more that you allow situations to dictate your reaction, the more dominance they gain over you life. The more dominance they gain over your life, the less control you 'experience' in your life. That "pattern" of behavior, which is NOT YOU, lives your life for you.

In martial arts, I would see this all the time on the mat and in the ring. Fighters would carry their baggage into the match and let that baggage determine the course of events. It's like they invited all of their fears into their body, possessing them like some demon incarnate. This creature – the culmination of all their fears – faces the opponent. Rarely, if ever, does the REAL PERSON arrive in the fight. S/he typically holds the back seat in their life, and pissed off that they cannot "do" anything about it.

I detect these fighters right away in the screening process. They are the ones blaming others and things for the events in their life, for their situation and conditions; they are their own victims because they forfeit control over their lives. They blame others for their piss poor performance because they don't realize that they COULD REGAIN CONTROL! If they realized this, then they would. Who wouldn't???

You must first realize that the "Pattern" of *Fear-Reactivity* is NOT YOU. You must disassociate with your past cycle of negative behavior. You are not your knee jerks. That phantom you will vanquish by regaining control of your life and by stepping up into the driver's seat and reclaiming your rightful position as caption of your Ship.

How do I know the difference between my authentic responses and my patterns of Fear-Reactivity?

Well, becoming aware of your knee jerks is certainly the first step. Recognizing the depth and breadth of those reactions will be humbling. So prepare for the pie! But it's not groveling about what you've become, because firstly, IT'S NOT YOU! Who you are is NOT that Pattern. You must disassociate with that pattern, distance yourself from mere habitual behavior.

In martial art, I named this *Differentiation*. Before you are able to see your performance for what it is, you must first be able to remove the filters from your perception of reality, remove the emotionalism from prejudicing your assessment of life. You must *Differentiate* between the Pattern and You.

It's only after *Differentiation* that you may go to the next step – *Integration*. And by next step, I don't mean that this happens globally throughout all decisions. It may happen in one direction of your life first; the easier, less stressful directions of your life first, in which you can more rapidly differentiate between *Fear-Reactivity* and the underlying You.

To differentiate however, you must first realize how you've IDENTIFIED with the *Fear-Reactivity*. The quintessential question when considering your body, *who is the YOU that purports to own your body which is not you?*

Of course the Body is an essential element of your personhood – just like your mind and your soul. You are a seamlessly contiguous and inextricably intertwined symphony of physical, mental and spiritual being. However, when you say "your body" you really allude to the Pattern – that which is not you.

Sounding really deep? Good! Depth does not mean inapplicable though. Remember that! How does this apply specifically?

Again... glad you asked. I'll tell you. Okay, so remember that your muscle tension, heart rate, blood pressure, breathing pattern (depth, frequency and quality) determine your hormonal arousal, which determines your emotional feelings, mental impression and eventually internal dialogue, or "thoughts?"

I could really expand on the process in scientific jargon (as my fans know I've done in the past.) However, it may get in the way for this book. This book isn't meant as an academic dissertation on psychophysiology. I have already created courses on that subject being used by psychologists worldwide, and truthfully, they're too meaty to DIRECTLY help the most people with their performance, health, strength, longevity, success, prosperity, et cetera. I intended for *Body-Flow* to immediately infuse you with enough information to understand the problem and create solutions... every day, right now, this second, out-of-the-package, first-read-through!

Let's just use the following as the architecture for exploring the impact upon your *Self-Image*... your image of your self, your impression of who you are, the 'thing' that you identify with as being "you."

23

WHAT HAPPENS BETWEEN AN EVENT AND MY REACTION TO IT?

I've alluded to the following process several times now. I named it *Stress Arousal Syndrome*. What you'll read next, well this entire book actually, involves the distillation of major portions of my experimentation and their implementation with my team of doctors and researchers in the realm of wellness, optimum human performance science and martial arts.

The *Stress Arousal Syndrome* is a step-by-step process of increasing alertness and mobilizing your total organism. It begins with monitoring and collecting information from the inside and from the outside environment. It continues to judge and evaluate the threat level of the information, and then elicits a reflex or reaction to address the stimulus.

The key words here are *reflex* and *reaction*. YOU are not involved in the process. You are not choosing to respond appropriately and with discernment to the issue. This is purely programming.

Stress, unfortunately, competes with awareness, and arousal interferes with response.

In motor science, your *Reaction* time is the length of time to become aware a stimulus. Your *Response* time is total length of time to observe, orient, decide and act upon the stimulus. If stress causes you to have difficulty becoming aware of and recognizing events, your total response time lengthens and becomes increasingly inaccurate.

Ever see a really stressed out person try to play tennis? The more and more frustrated she becomes, the greater her reaction time becomes to become aware of and recognize returns, and the longer and longer it takes for her to respond, if at all.

I use *Response* here to relate to the difference between reacting to noise and responding to the actual signal (the message within all the ambient junk). For instance, if you open a door to a loud room, because you needed to quickly hear your friend's answer to a question you had asked him to go in and yell back to you, the "noise" would be all of the din of the room, and the signal would be his one voice and the message it contained (the answer you were waiting to hear.) You could react to all of the noise by becoming stressed, straining to tune out everything but your friend's voice, or you could reflexively shrink back at the sudden sonic boom of noise emanating from the room.

Reflexes are those actions that are hard-wired into you – the signal never gets to your brain, because it's programmed to act at the spinal level. You don't need to think to pull your hand off a hot burner. Reflexes are helpful jump-starts out of dangerous situations.

Reactions are learned and conditioned actions bound to a general stimulus. Imagine standing at the edge of a tennis court. You have a little experience, but you're facing Chris Evert. Chris serves directly at you. The ball steams across the court about as fast as rubber can fly. Instead of maneuvering for a return, the speed is so overwhelming, the stress so high that your arms come up to protect your head, your knees bend and you duck, clenching your teeth and eyes shut. You never have a chance to access your skills, because the fearful reactions competed AND WON for dominance in motor action.

Or to return to the "loud room" analogy, your reaction could be to shout over your friend's voice yelling at him to just return outside with you. You could have discerned what he said through paying attention to the "signal" but your reaction was frustration.

These reactions are learned and conditioned every moment of your life, ever time that you permit the "inner gremlin" to steer the Vehicle on the path of your life. By understanding this process, you will be able to identify that which is not you, your Patterned *Fear-Reactivity*, and as a result uncover that which is you: your natural talent, genius and abundance. As a result, you will unbind your flow to reveal your birthright to *Body-Flow*.

WHAT IS THE STRESS AROUSAL SYNDROME PROCESS?

The SAS comprises the following capacities step-by-step:

1. *Movement* This involves all temporal and spatial changes in the configuration of your living ("somatic") body and its parts, such as breathing, eating, speaking, blood circulation, and digestion. This is your moment-to-moment state that your body evaluates and which is the platform from which you interface with the environment.

Notice I wrote STATE and not TRAIT. A state is what happens, and if repeated, adapted to and progressed upon; whereas, a "trait" is what it becomes as a (quasi)-permanent behavior. When I write "Patterns of *Fear-Reactivity*" I'm speaking to the network of traits with whom you have identified as "you" – such as I or *"so and so makes me so angry that I just fly off the handle whenever s/he says _____."* Those judgments are the culmination of conditioning STATES, just like any skill.

Everything is a skill, be it fatness or fitness, fear or anger, sorrow or frustration. The good news is that at any time, you can choose to not reinforce a particular STATE by changing your behavior. You can choose which TRAITS you cultivate. And it begins here, with Movement, the most fundamental aspect of a living ("somatic") bodily existence.

2. *Sensation* What you sense you receive from two inputs: from the Extroceptive (the "five senses") and from the Interoceptive (the *Sixth Sense: Proprioception* and *Vestibular Sense*). I shall discus the *Sixth Sense* in the next section, which includes pain, spatial orientation, time passage, rhythm, force/pressure, velocity/acceleration, weight/gravity, balance/equilibrium and stabilization.

Basically, think of this as the information-gathering phase where you reconnoiter and monitor events as they transpire in the world around and within. Probably this is the LEAST understood aspect of this process and accounts for several centuries of blundering in Western Philosophy.

Once you understand how you GATHER information then you will gain the ability to FILTER the noise in order to AMPLIFY true signals. Think of your brain as a satellite dish – you can direct the reception to collect critical data, and you can tune out the noise. Think of noise as like ambient information which does not contribute to your development as a person: your transcendence beyond your old Patterns of *Fear-Reactivity*. Like the old Russian saying, *"the man may be the head of the family, but the woman is the neck. She can turn the head to pay attention to whatever she wishes."* You learn to turn the satellite dish to find the clearest signal of crucial information.

The best book on this subject is a frighteningly intimidating textbook edited by Scott M. Lephart and Freddie H. Fu entitled, <u>*Proprioception and Neuromuscular Control in Joint Stability*</u>.

3. *Emotions* This step is actually divided into three sub-steps, and really, for brevity's sake, there's no reason that we need to get very technical when it comes to Stress Physiology. Many of my fans know how jargonized this field rapidly becomes. I want to

streamline this and make it totally accessible to everyone so let's look at the following process.

To understand what emotions are, you need to realize that people often inappropriately interchange "feelings" for "emotions." Feelings are only one sub-set of emotions. And because of the basic misuse of the terms, people think that emotions are some wild mustang that lay outside of their control. Feelings are rooted concretely in your movement... the first step, remember? And they begin with Autonomic arousal:

Autonomic: This capacity provides quick mobilization of energy for vigorous movement, such as increased heart rate, blood pressure, muscular tension, respiration, core temperature, & pupil dilation.

Hormonal: When the Autonomic does not suffice to accomplish fight or flight, this capacity reinforces it by washing the system with a supercharged chemical cocktail including epinephrine, norepinephrine, aldosterone, endorphins, etc.

One major problem here regards the rate at which this fuel injection occurs. If you face numerous, intense, frequent, and/or complex stressors, then these chemicals are not slowly added to your system. You immediately go into RED-ALERT survival mode, and involuntarily you throw the sluice gate wide open and DUMP all these chemicals undiluted, full-strength into your system. It throws your system into total _Shock_ – which is actually the appropriate scientific term.

Another danger here is that if you fail to resolve the threat, if you fail to fight or flee, if you become tolerant to higher and higher levels of stress, the chemical released to halt your internal alarm system does not suffice to shut down your arousal. You fall prey to _Tonic Immobility_, as well as facing _Post-Traumatic Stress Disorder_, _Chronic Fatigue_, etc.

As I've written earlier, there are major dangers here for your health, performance and strength, but the worst, arguably, is the impact this has upon _Self-Image_. This is directly the ROOT of all of the stress-related illnesses and diseases.

The best book on this subject is a rather daunting textbook by Robert M. Sapolsky entitled, _Why Zebras Don't Get Ulcers_.

Feelings: This is the brain's interpretation of sensory feedback from the muscles and organs that produce the reactions. This feedback constitutes what it is to call "your feelings." Familiar emotions include joy, grief, anger, self-respect, inferiority, super-sensitivity, and other conscious and unconscious emotions. You are not the feelings that erupt from arousal and hyper-arousal. Who you are lies beneath your Patterns of **Fear-Reactivity**.

The best book on this subject is a rather daunting textbook by David H. Barlow entitled, _Anxiety and Its Disorders_ (2nd Edition).

4. **Thoughts** This step is actually broken into two sub-steps:

Mental Impressions: This relates to memory in that you anchor certain feelings together, and you access those related emotions when you confront a similar experience. This accounts for the host of Bodywork methods in the industry in that if you overcome a similar task, you often "free the feelings" from a passed suppressed, unaddressed event.

<u>Self-Dialogue</u>: This capacity acts as the function of the intellect, such as understanding, classifications, imagination, and memory. Thoughts erupt from feelings.

Probably the entire discipline of Western Philosophy from Ancient Greece to the present remained locked within this ephemeral quicksand, sinking with every attempt to swim ashore, spending most of their time thinking themselves deeper and deeper into non-Sensical conclusions. Without understanding that how you feel determines your thoughts, without understanding that your thoughts, your very self-image are a product of concrete physical processes, you become lost – *a ghost in the machine.*

Being a fighter, I had little use for intangibles. For me, will was going an extra round, soul was enduring another blow, spirit was facing the next foe. If what I thought interfered with my ability to triumph over my opponent, I "changed my mind." Having the luxury of true threats, of humans meaning me actual bodily harm, and engaged in hand to hand combat, I was fortunate enough to learn rapidly what contributed to development and what hampered it.

I say "luxury" not with tongue in cheek. I spent many years in the University observing my classmates in course after course of "advanced" Philosophy. I know first hand that you can't think your way out of a crisis. That life regards pragmatic solutions, not idle pontification.

Thoughts… plain and simple are the product of your Movement.

The best book on this subject is a VERY accessible (though out of print) book introducing some of the basic *Peak Performance* techniques that I studied in the former Soviet Union with their Olympic and National Coaching staff, and the trainers of their special military operations and secret police. The book written by Grigori Raiport entitled - *Red Gold*. For the most thorough and well-packaged presentation on peak performance for combat (whether on the battlefield or in the board room), I also suggest *Flow-State Performance Spiral* and *Flow-Fighting* published by yours truly at RMAX.tv Productions www.RMAX.tv.

Separating the above capacities in **Stress Arousal Syndrome** is a function of speech alone<u>!</u> It is impossible <u>in reality</u> to separate them. It follows from this interaction that *detailed attention to any one capacity necessarily influences the others* – the whole person and your self-image. In reality there is no practical way of correcting an individual except through incremental progression alternating between whole and its parts.

OTHERS AND YOUR PATTERNS OF FEAR-REACTIVITY

Physical discipline seems to "transform" people. Friends and family pose great resistance to changes. They often have difficulty accepting transformations in people, because though you changed, they remained the same, and do not understand who this "new you" is. Changes in posture, eating behavior, coordination, grace, any development in motor skill pose a 'threat' to the "person" whom others have come to identify as "you." THEY ASSOCIATE THE PATTERNS WITH WHO THEY THINK YOU ARE!

This is why change is hard. It's not only the transcendence from your Patterns of **_Fear-Reactivity_**, but facing the ubiquitous resistance of reinforced association of your past reactions with who you are. You spent a great deal of time teaching people to think that you were those reactions. You spent all that time letting people "get to know" that cycle of behavior, so they believe you are it. They think you are, what you were.

But just like you will overcome, and leverage out that doppelganger who purports to be you, so too will your friends and family eventually come to learn who it is that you really are.

Don't worry. True friends and real family stick around, because intuitively they've always known who you **really** are, and **loved** you for it. And because they're true friends and real family, they've always wanted you to transcend those old, negative patterns.

Bottom line? If they don't want you to shine, if they resist your "becoming," if they attempt to stifle you transcending your addictions and attachments, remember to have compassion for them – for they too have identified with their Patterns… and you too may have associated their Patterns with who they really are.

Do you really see THEM for who they truly are… or are you just attending their reactions? Do you just anticipate how they will react to situations and events and purport to know "them?"

It's that anticipation of how a person will react which is what it is to associate someone with their negative anchors on their performance, health, strength… and personhood.

LIFE'S MOST HAZARDOUS ADDICTION: SELF-IMAGE

The strongest addiction in humanity is addiction to self-image. Remember, the image of the self here I refer to regards the network of Patterned *Fear-Reactivity* – the things that people anticipate you will do, how they expect you to behave, the reactions you've taught them you shall have.

We all know spontaneity, creativity, improvisation, innovation… yet few of us LIVE it. We knew it in our formative years. We "played" constantly. How many of you still do? How many of you are willing to risk <u>what</u> you are for who you could **become**? Do you willing embrace the possibility of embarrassment? Heck, if there's something that you suspect may embarrass you, that's a signpost stating, *"BEWARE! Here is something you ought to pay attention to! Here is a lesson!"*

You face great resistance in transcending past patterns. The old self that you wear becomes like a heavy, rusty suit of plate-mail armor. And some people just keep grabbing more pieces they stumble upon, making that fortress impenetrable… but also inescapable.

You forget what you look like under that armor of tension and prejudice, malice and frustration, embarrassment and anxiety. You forget what it was like to be free, to move and dance, and spring and sprint, to play like a babe, to climb trees, to fight like an animal, to make love with reckless abandon, to roll in the dirt, to wrestle with a friend, to learn a new instrument, or ride a new toy. All that armor does is slow you down, and eventually with enough tears and sweat, you rust shut, and shutdown. Immobile. Imprisoned by your solidified *Fear-Reactivity*.

If those thoughts, if that internal dialogue – that "person" that speaks to you and passes judgment on things you do and events you see, hear, taste, touch and smell (and intuit), that person has BECOME that armor. That person, who flies of the handle, turns down an opportunity to try something new or take a risk; that person who reluctantly backs away from learning a new craft or introducing themselves to a new person; that person is <u>not you</u>.

It is just a cunning complex of fears. You **can choose** to ACT otherwise. You can experience hesitation and choose to smirk and dash forward into the unknown, to pick up your machete and pioneer your own path, beat your drum your own damn way, *thank you very much!*

That voice though, those fears, vie for existence. 'It' (the collective entangled mass of those fears) attempts "self-preservation" and tells you that you're inadequate, incompetent, too fat, too old, too young, too much of a girl, too complex, too cultured, too elite, too inexperienced, too tired, too hungry, too ill-prepared, too, too, too… ad nauseum.

Listen to it, then smile, for it is <u>not you</u>. Relax, and be comfortable with the little gremlin who attempts to fool you. You can choose to interrupt those patterns. You can, quite instantly, move a different direction, without a "reason" to explain to the mind-hobgoblins.

Remember those tensions dump hormones, which produce feelings, which create thoughts. The patterns of tensions create thoughts! You can cut the disease off at the root. You can decapitate the old self by moving differently. It's not going to be easy. And you'll confront all those Fear-Reactive patterns as you move outside your "comfort zone" – the realm of expected, anticipated movement.

We grow addicted to limitation. We grow "comfortable." We fortify and even actively attack potential challenges to our "comfort zone" – which comprise the defined boundaries of your image of your self. Not who you are, but who you think you are not, what you think you should not be capable of, or what you should not be defined as.

We become addicted to that nice little castle and we ensure that we never invite guests who will challenge the little fiefdom we each call "The Kingdom of Me."

You can overcome this addiction. You can emancipate yourself from being a self-junky. You can become self-less, and as a result liberate your natural talent, genius and abundance.

Your movement, structural alignment (such as your posture and carriage and gait)), your breathing and heart rate and blood pressure, as a total package, create your thoughts – that inner narrator who speaks to you. You're going to meet great resistance as you exceed the limitations of those patterns. But first you need to realize that although the Path is an internal one, your existence occurs in the external world.

The greatest resistance you shall meet for transcending your self-image, comes from those closest to you – your friends and family, and then, of course... your self (the closest)... who shall attempt to defend its existence like any creature.

When you change how you carry yourself, how you stand, how you sit, move, fight, play, speak, dress, you break the social contract with friends and family who are locked within them selves. Those people who enable your addictions, who contribute to your self-abuse, will REACT to oppose your changes (for it indeed threatens their self status quo!) They will chastise you, attempt to embarrass you, and even outright violently attempt to prohibit you from changing.

Transcending your self-image separates you from inauthentic relationships. Only the true friends and real family will remain. These are the people that have seen through your veneer, seen through the illusion of your patterned reactivity, seen through your fears, doubts, hesitations. They attempt at all costs to "Lift you Up" out of those fettering patterns. They know and resonate with your INTEGRITY – that which is INTEGRAL to you, rather than that which is not you – your *Fear-Reactivity*.

And in truth, few people if any Walk with you throughout your entire life. You need to look at people in your life as blessed guests, welcomed visitors. People, who visit for an extended duration, say your entire life, well... they will only be those people who not only support and help lift-up who YOU are, but they are on the Path too of transcending them selves.

If you view these fellow seekers, who are constantly off doing "the work" – playing, taking risks, being life-adventurers, you appreciate them, never take them for granted, and if you haven't seen them for years, it's as if you were never apart. If you view them as welcomed visitors, you will never attempt to define them, pigeonhole and compartmentalize who they truly are. You never associate them with their failures, and never enable them to identify with the fears they seek to confront and overcome.

You can do this. You can overcome the addiction, and even help others overcome their own. Like any addiction, it requires vigilance and practice.

Life is one endless sequence of decisions, and even if you've been doing the same cancerous thing your entire life, one day, right now, you can just CHOOSE otherwise.

Once down that Path, you may falter, you may drop back into your Patterns of *Fear-Reactivity*, you may hear that gremlin climbing back trying to regain a foothold on your behavior, but with persistence and determination, and armed with the confidence that there is a nation of other seekers striving valiantly against limitation, mediocrity and disease, you can get up, dust off, and dare to again choose otherwise.

In this quest to transcend your self-image, you are often a lone traveler. But as I've said many places, **<u>although you may be a lone traveler, we are all alone in this together</u>**.

VICTIMIZATION BY THE SELF

Ultimately, the resistance is ONLY within you – you either resist flow (***Residual Muscle Tension***), or you've forgotten how to flow (***Sensory Motor Amnesia***).

However, thoughts arise blaming others for your situation, attributing others with accountability for your condition and situation.

With martial artists, pro athletes, soldiers, even business tycoons, I encounter this all the time in private sessions. It's like recording a laundry list of everyone else in the world responsible for his or her shortcomings. "That damn referee!" one fighter complains; "inappropriate governmental sanctions from such-and-such Senator who pockets our taxes to fund his yada, yada, yada…" Or worse come the excuses of those who are abused by others, "he won't let me; he doesn't like when I stand up like 'a man' he says." They fill volumes of journals of grievances against others, and they do not realize UNTIL THEY CHOOSE TO CHANGE THEIR SELF-IMAGE that they were **always and already in control**.

You are <u>always and already masterful, graceful, powerful</u>. You need to realize this, **right now**. The whole purpose of this book helps you leverage out your *Bound-Flow*.

But you need to first take responsibility, <u>accept full accountability</u> for your ACTIONS. And that's all they are… those negative thoughts, that idle abusive chatter in your head – they are phantoms, wraiths, gremlins, hobgoblins... illusionary monsters under the bed. You can bring light to that dark closet. You can vanquish the apparitions. But you need to stop being the Victim of your self – the collective patterns of *Fear-Reactivity*.

I see fighters hemorrhaging performance all the time – their fears, hesitations, doubts, all sap their energy, slow their movement and inhibit their potential. It's sad to observe, because they do not take responsibility for their actions. It's the fault of the referee's call, the crowd's noise, the bad food for breakfast, the girlfriend's/boyfriend's argument, the coach's methods, the quality of the shoes, the length of the rounds, the chill in the weather, blah, blah, blah… endlessly. They don't realize that the desire to attach others with control over their lives relinquishes their control. By blaming others, you FORFEIT your God-given RIGHT to pilot your life!

Remember that pernicious little banter in your head is <u>not you</u>, but only you can change it. That inner dialogue is a process beginning from how you respond to the events in your life as they unfold. So you can thwart their existence, rip the proverbial rug out from underneath them so they have nothing upon which to stand… by changing your physical being.

It IS that simple, though it shall be difficult and painful. Tearing down the walls will always be painful. And remember that as you do, you shall become more vulnerable, you shall increase your sensitivity to events. But that's not a bad thing. Before you can outmaneuver resistance, before you can regain your Mastery over the self, you need to first tear down the patterns, tear down the walls.

HOW DO I GET FREE FROM MY FEAR-REACTIVITY?

Since the nervous system is occupied mainly with movement, emotional reactions and negative internal dialogue can be modified by experience.

Self-image consists of a pattern of reactions interacting with the environment, so CHOOSING to respond, rather than being enslaved to *Fear-Reactivity* liberates you from the limitations of an image of self, returns autonomy to your life, reclaims your rightful control over your performance, strength and health.

If you reference the *Stress Arousal Syndrome*, you find that the first step in all negative dialogue, in all rampant feelings, regards movement, structural alignment and breathing. Impacting any of these elements necessarily influences self-image, unbinds flow; just as allowing fear to embed a reaction creates a negative self-image, binds flow.

Basically, if you remember after sensations comes the autonomic – muscle tension, heart rate, blood pressure, breathing behavior. Well, this is the first evidence you receive. It's the first blip on the radar.

Think of it this way. Almost a decade ago, I started explaining it to people that fear, trauma, stress… dis-integrates your breathing, movement, and structural alignment. When you're anxious, your breathing becomes shallow and rapid, right? When you're pissed out of your mind, furious, you often hold your breath, right? When you're exasperated and frustrated you often sigh and growl, right? And when you're anxious, angry or frustrated, how do your muscles tense, how do your carry yourself, how does your heartbeat and your blood pressure vary?

Fear, trauma, and stress break down, or as I like to point out, dis-integrate your breathing, movement and structure. Dis-integrate. They are integrated by natural function. When things in your life go well, you seem to just run like a river right – you breath perfectly in sync with your movements and you carry yourself like an anti-gravitational master!

This is why, unknowingly, physical disciplines such as Yoga, Tai Chi and Zdorovye bring peace back to the frenetic lifestyle of so many people. It's the only time in their day when they return to the way they were designed to function – with their breathing, movements and alignment properly integrated.

But how frustrating those classes can be for so many people who try to gain the flow of the Masters! They watch with cognitive dissonance trying to understand how the Masters "learned" such grace and poise and power. It baffles them. Why? Because they think that the Masters LEARNED grace and poise and power.

Grace and poise and power are your birthright!!! It's the way you naturally function. It's what you're designed to do IF you would only get out of your own way, if you would only stop dis-integrating your breathing, movement and structure by reacting to stress, trauma and fear.

Easier said than done, eh? You bet! That's why we need some Daily Personal Practice to deepen our choices, to sophisticate the connection of mind, body and spirit, to groove flow by getting out of its way and just cruising.

The difficulty of these disciplines is that they are typically taught by a person attempting to impose the process that they underwent to unbind their flow. One emphasizes breathing as the essential task. Another emphasized movement, and still another – structural alignment.

Well, they're all wrong. None are the essential task – but rather they ALL are. It depends upon the situation. If you're having difficulty with your breathing, you can focus upon your movement and your structure. If you're encountering a problem with your movement, you can focus upon your structure and your breathing. And if you've discovered a problem with your structure, you can focus on your breathing and your movement. They are each tools. If you have trouble with one, the other two combined will unlock the puzzle.

I've said this for a long time, and it's probably the most often quoted of my work:

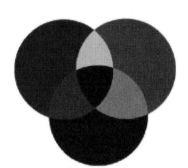

Breathing + Structure creates Movement

Movement + Breathing creates Structure

Structure + Movement creates Breathing

As you can see in the illustration to the right: breathing, movement and structure directly influence each other, and all three integrated produce... *Body-Flow*.

When you find a "lock" in your breathing, movement or structure, you can unbind flow, by assembling the performance goals of the other two. It's a simple, yet an increasingly, infinitely sophisticated process of discovery.

You reclaim *Body-Flow* by re-integrating breathing, movement, and structure. Your task is to explore my unique exercises that I have designed and selected to challenge you and to liberate you. Each new exercise is a puzzle. You will travel through the puzzle and come to a blocked path – some element of *Bound-Flow* within you. You need to retrace your steps, and like an alchemist compose a new brew to cure yourself of that binding. The above formula will provide you with a Legend to the Map.

Next, I'll describe the Map, so that you can begin to navigate the Landscape, which is your unlimited talent, genius and abundance.

GOING DEEPLY: MY JOURNEY CREATING BODY-FLOW

The former USSR conducted extensive research into the Sixth Sense, often dressing the research as "paranormal investigation" to propagandize foreigners into fear of Soviet occult powers. Now of course we have every recent émigré attempting to play off those decades of Cold War and bottle their crazy for the low, low price of… whatever they can charge by Remote Viewing your bank account. It's deplorable, but as long as people want short cuts, they'll buy videos on psychic fireballs.

My entire experience with this business has been a seemingly endless sequence of discovering the sleight of hand behind the "magic." Each of them scrambling for some rationalization – he wasn't ready; it doesn't work on trained fighters; it's unethical to show Randi; yada, yada, yada.

Why does it always have to be cloaked in such woo-woo non-Sense? Why can't Nature be AMAZING enough and Life MYSTERIOUS enough without needing to deceive people?

I remember a time when I was "invited" (read here – challenged) to visit a particular Jiu-jitsu school because of the instructors had a secret beef with me. He thought that he would have an advantage by getting me on his block. Little did he realize that he had MORE to lose by my presence in his school: he would lose face if he lost to someone of whom he had spoken ill. When I did arrive, I had to "run the line" fighting everyone in the school from lowest ranked to highest, and all the instructors.

I used the same trick on all of them, because I knew that with each successful attempt, the upper ranks would focus all their mental preparation on thwarting that one maneuver. Little did they realize that I had won, simply by this, by getting them to fixate on one thing. There are an infinite number of set-ups to any particular maneuver. If they fixated on the maneuver, they would never see the set-up.

After cleaning the house and facing the head instructor, he asked to go several times insisting that he was not prepared, until after many flight lessons and many sharp introductions to the mat, he submitted. In private, this particular instructor said that my "energy" was too far developed for him to stop with "mere physical technique." I shook his hand and shook my head. There was no way to argue with his ego, so I left him in the hopes that he would one day (perhaps by reading this) know that there are no secret powers… just daily deepening of personal practice.

There seems to be no end to playing upon peoples *Fear-Reactivity*, and the Cold War produced a great many victims. Propaganda aside, however, the former Soviet Union developed and applied methods that gained success in all international sports. Russian sport scientist and authority Dr. Michael Yessis explains, *"To develop fitness programs for both the public and serious athletes, hundreds of scientists in the USSR are involved in full-time research into all aspects of physical well-being. At the National Research Institute of Physical Culture in Moscow, for instance, the 'Department of Maximology' conducts studies primarily on the nation's elite athletes, with the help of an array of sophisticated equipment in its laboratories, and develops new methods of strength and power training and techniques for psychological preparation for competition."*

Outside the walls of the _Department of Maximology_, few Soviet citizens knew the nature of this research combining the academic fields of sport psychology, stress physiology, and biomechanics. Because these methods were implemented for the space and defense programs, the research was locked under a stamp of *"Absolute Secrecy."*

I found the severity level of this secrecy, when I fought a Russian Master of Sport in SAMBO who was also the Chief of Hand-to-Hand Combat for Russia's largest and most famous space-launching site – Baikanor.

My staff filmed the exhibition fight. We were "advised" later that we did not have permission to release the footage because it included images of the chief trainer and of the special maneuvers he attempted to apply. I had been instructed by the same principles, so I found this strange. I even defeated my opponent, something never before heard of for an American. Nonetheless, it seems the fingers of propaganda stretch far and grip strongly.

To the best of my understanding, this paranoia stems from the fact that the <u>Committee for Physical Culture and Sports</u>, the umbrella organ regulating all athletic activities in the former Soviet Union, was not an adjunct to any ministry such as health or education. Its functionaries reported exclusively and directly to the <u>Department of Propaganda</u> itself. To say this in another way, this Soviet research into elite performance held the primary function of promoting the USSR and the Communist way of life. Athletics served a two-pronged function in the Soviet Union: on one side, it promoted the military preparedness of every able citizen, and on the other side, it demonstrated to the world the alleged supremacy of Communist society.

Billions of dollars were invested in this research, which Westerners are only now beginning to implement. I used that information to win international championships and defeat them at their own form of combat called SAMBO – a Russian acronym for "unarmed self-defense." It's a brutal fighting form – the only one I know of where if you break your opponent's limbs, you win.

That was many years ago, and tens of thousands of cumulative hours of testing ago. This is the primary reason that I intended to compile and refine this research through RMAX.tv Productions. Now, my courses have helped more champions from more martial art styles achieve greatness than anyone in history as well as thousands upon thousands of athletes and enthusiasts from across the world.

What now seems the trend, the edge, or the innovative in the field today can be, in part or in whole, traced back to this pool of research conducted in my department at RMAX.tv Productions – the _Life Enhancement Solutions_. People love to debate this fact. I choose to capitalize on the research and discoveries and move forward to help American athletes and military personnel, and the public at large.

The Soviet Union pursued a pragmatic approach to athletics. Only results mattered. No ego would be tolerated – no personal agendas, no private benefit, no individual aspiration. The exclusive goal was to optimize performance of Soviet athletics for the glory of the Communist system. This research began in the 1920's in order to prepare for the Olympic Games, which the Soviet Union would enter post-Tsarist Russia (1924).

The Soviets discovered that there is no basic difference between the psychological requirements of an athlete and that of a jet-fighter pilot or cosmonaut. To discover the outer limits of human performance, the Soviets researched deeply into the *Trinity* of the somatic (or "living body") experience: the physical, the mental, and the emotional. They pushed the envelope of optimal performance through specialized techniques developed and proven in athletic competition and combative engagements.

In the Soviet Union, coaches learned and applied methods of massage, postural manipulation, and physical exercise specifically to optimize the Sixth Sense in athletes, soldiers and even citizenry. Descriptions of these techniques appear in various Russian sport science publications, such as *Theory and Practice of Physical Culture*. Soviet sport science research found revitalization in modern Russia with the *RETAL: Russian Combat Skill Consultant Scientific & Practical Training Center* – the Russian research laboratory for the ROSS Training System. The specialized conditioning strategies devised in these secret State labs led the USSR and today's Russia to countless triumphs in Olympic sports performance, as well as to frightening motor perfection of their elite military special operations units (the *Spetsnaz*).

Russian sports scientists, such as Dr. Mel Siff and Dr. Yuri Verkhoshansky, insist that this type of training is crucial and neglected in conventional sports methods:

"Strength, efficiency and safety of movement is determined primarily by neuromuscular factors, in particular the sense of kinesthesia and the underlying proprioceptive mechanisms which inform us about where all the components of our musculoskeletal system are and what they are doing relative to one another in space and time. The integration of information from all the other senses, together with this proprioceptive information enables us to execute a given movement in the most appropriate way in terms of pattern, velocity, acceleration and timing. This involves coordination of eye-hand, eye-foot or body-apparatus, processes that receive a great deal of attention in technical training. Inadequate time, however, is generally devoted to specific training of proprioception, even though its importance is central to physiotherapy rehabilitation system known as PNF (Proprioceptive Neuromuscular Facilitation)" (*Supertraining*).

Understanding what was TRULY researched and discovered in the former Soviet Union directly from the Olympic coaches and the personnel who trained the military special forces instructors provided me with a unique opportunity to explain the "Sixth Sense" in easy to understand, totally accessible terms. More importantly, this book will allow you to ACCELERATE your ability to access that latent talent, genius and abundance within you!

WHAT IS THE SIXTH SENSE?

People conventionally understand Exteroceptive - the five senses of hearing, touching, seeing, tasting, and smelling. But many people discuss the nature of the *Sixth-Sense* as extra-sensory perception – sensing beyond the senses. Perhaps they are correct that it is beyond the five senses, but it is not beyond sense. In other words, the Sixth Sense is not non-sense – it is very much sensory perception. It's Interoceptive. If anything, **Body-Flow** introduces **the ONLY true No Non-Sense Approach**.

People see the nimble power, uncanny accuracy, and bewildering intuition of martial art masters and presume them to be keepers of esoteric powers. Masters of various internal martial art styles have developed elaborate theories and convoluted programs to develop the Sixth Sense. Many are charlatans, many of them have no idea and as a result craft various "tricks" to impress and entertain crowds. But they are false prophets preaching crazy. This is the main reason why martial arts before this book never had access to being assimilated into a rational, scientific perspective. *Because of the non-sense.*

Occam's Razor states, *"one should not increase, beyond the necessary, the number of entities required to explain anything"* or, in other words: all things being equal, the simplest solution among several possible solutions to a given problem is the "best" one.

What is the simplest explanation of the Sixth Sense and how to develop it? The best and most obvious answer is that the Sixth Sense is the *Proprioception* – the refinement of bodily awareness in time and space.

WHAT IS PROPRIOCEPTION?

Pencil-pushing "Experts" still remain locked in a struggle to define this question ever since Sherrington coined the term in 1906. Proprioception very succinctly, though not very simply, involves all those inputs which originate from the joints, muscles, tendons and deep tissue, and those signals sent to your Central Nervous System for processing.

Proprioception has nothing to do with your CNS' processing of this information, nor does it have anything to do with reflexes, reactions and responses. It's a SENSE. It's how you perceive your place in the world, because it directly assesses your muscular tensions (including your movements and respiratory control), postural equilibrium, and joint stability.

Proprioception gathers this information through special sensors in your muscles, connective tissues, and joints. Like satellite dishes dedicated to different channels, there are five different "receptions":

- Nociceptors detect levels of pain, aches, trauma in the body

- Chemoreceptors detect changes in internal and external chemistry, such as alluded to above with hormonal arousal in the *Stress Arousal Syndrome*.

- Electro-magnetic receptors detect changes in the electromagnetic field in which we live, and accounts for the host of "energy work" disciplines that evolved over millennia. Only recently, however, has the rational, scientific community arrived at a level of sophistication where it can understand these energy-work disciplines.

- Thermoreceptors – detect changes in temperature, externally and internally.

- Mechanoreceptors – detects three different though similar categories of information:

    o *Position Sense*, also known as "joint sense" detects the position of all of your joints in three dimensional space; including postural equilibrium, joint stability

    o *Movement Sense*, also known as "kinesthetic sense" detects all of the changes in velocity, direction, and angle of all of your movement.

    o *Tension Sense*, also known as "force sense" which detects all of the levels, changes, and rates of tension in your muscles, tendons and ligaments, as well as pressure and vibration.

All of this information is received and converted into a final common signal that is transmitted to your CNS. Think about this now. The Sixth Sense is the amalgam of all of the above processed simultaneously and transmitted to your brain to process, and then decide on how to interact with the environment. It's such an amazing system!

But let's look at something here. Let's consider where in the game you collect this information. Your nervous system can basically be divided into three parts. Let's look at them in reverse order from farthest from the brain to nearest:

Spinal Cord receives the proprioceptive information.

Brain Stem receives visual (your eyes) and vestibular information: the fluid gyroscope in your inner ear which senses position, velocity, and acceleration of the head in relation to the body and acts as an internal guidance and balance system. A lot of bodywork methods deal with this calling it "Primary Control" but as you can see, it's not the earliest player in collecting information.

Cerebral Cortex processes all the sensory information and forms an internal representation of all of it. I call this your *Mental Blueprint*: essential information for your brain integrated it into a moment-to-moment portrait of your movement in relation to your environment. What's very important to understand here is that your Mental Blueprint is the brain's interpretive model of your physical Self-Image (referred to in *The Matrix* by *Morpheus* as "Residual Self-Image").

Mental Blueprint and Self-Image

As a whole, these physiological data collectors create an ongoing, moment-to-moment report of your bodily status in your brain, your *Mental Blueprint*. This entire process relays very accurate information about what your body does, but more importantly who you are – your *Self-Image*. Once it is communicated, your brain takes the sensory information and renders a three-dimensional portrait of you in your environment. This *Mental Blueprint* changes from each moment to the next.

The *Sixth Sense*, Proprioception, is so powerful that it causes the most widespread and intense electrical activity in the brain. For example, using your mental blueprint you can differentiate between two disparate arm positions that are greater than 1.25 centimeters apart.

It's the *Mental Blueprint* which permits you to close your eyes and touch your nose – the popular sobriety test. It's a small task, but absolutely amazing to consider. The *Mental Blueprint* is an internal sensory schema of everything in your environment. Sit down, close your fist, and try and touch your friend's nose. Start fast, but slow down to just a touch. You're friend will be glad that you got it correct on the first try! Successfully projecting the trajectory of his nose involves a highly sophisticated symphony of muscle, bone and connective tissue.

I like to explain to people what the *Mental Blueprint* is by demonstrating what happens when you don't have it. The *APA Monitor* (Azar, 1998) reported a case where a man, because of a certain viral infection, had lost his kinesthesia – his ability to internally represent bodily position in space. Despite the fact that all of his motor functions were fine, if you removed his sight, he could not even stand! He compensated after significant years of trial and error and managed to walk and move with relative competence. However, should anyone come into the room and turn of the lights, he would immediately fall to the floor in a heap, being able to get up only if someone turned on the lights.

Without his vision he had no "frame of reference" (*Mental Blueprint*) on where to place his hands down on the floor, how to elevate his elbow over hand with a sufficient angle to leverage himself off the floor. When standing, deprived of vision, he had no cues on where to place his feet underneath his center of gravity, no cues on how to shift his weight, no cues on how to maintain his balance. This was a rare case, but it definitely demonstrates the impact of just one subsection of Proprioception... the *Sixth Sense*.

However, we allow the other information to compete and dominate our information collecting.

YOUR THRESHOLD OF PAIN = YOUR THRESHOLD OF PERFORMANCE

People have heard me say this in many places. However, it's rarely understood. When I say your pain threshold determines your performance levels, I refer to the fact that *pain competes for your performance.*

For instance, the signal which is capable of dominating all of the other channels is Nociception. Pain, ache, and trauma override the other signals due to the urgency of the message to arrive at the CNS. This is simply an evolutionarily stable survival strategy. If we didn't get this information to our brains so that we could process it and DO something about it immediately, well… we wouldn't have survived this long as a species, now would we?

The problem from a motor skill development perspective is that the presence of pain, aches and trauma COMPETE with your ability to unlock your potential. I see this all the time with my cadre of meathead fighters who would rather beat each other Sense-less in sparring rather than working on the sophisticating their performance. They fail to realize, because of ego, that pain, aches and trauma override the other information coming in… Why do you think so few fighters are graceful, masterful? Why do only a few "natural athletes" evolve? Why do you think that there are some so-called "flukes" who become just awe-inspiring demons of efficiency? Why are there so few people who develop the technical wizardry of the Greats?

Well, the answer's simple: incorrect training methods and protocol. You can't uncover your **Body-Flow** by inducing pain, aches and trauma – **Fear-Reactivity**. You must do the opposite.

With all of my clients who are martial art coaches and fighters from various styles, I teach them a concept I coined called *Soft-Work*. Basically *Soft-Work* is all of the complexity of fighting without the pain. This catapults their abilities because of it amplifies the Mechanoreceptive signal.

If you're only doing *Toughness Training* (or as I call it in martial art – *Hard-Work*), you'll increase how much you can endure, how much pain you can take, how much shock you can absorb, but you won't be improving your technical sensitivity, coordination, agility, balance. Basically, you won't refine your skills. Just look at how goofy and stiff most fighters are, most athletes for that matter. Only a rare few display that essential grace and masterful motion that we call athletic beauty.

If you're an athlete, you must balance *Hard-Work* (how effective you are) and *Soft-Work* (how efficient you are). But for ALL people, in your daily life, you may work very hard at your vocation, you may work very hard in your home life, you may work very hard in your personal training, but can you work softly? Can you refine your efficiency with the most sophisticated tool you control? That tool of course is YOU!

If you're constantly living in pain, with aches and experiencing trauma (or not resolving past trauma), then how do you expect to unlock your talent, genius and abundance? How do you expect to reclaim your **Body-Flow**? Working hard in life is a necessary, but insufficient component of masterful existence!

You can't stop to pain, the aches, the trauma, but you can unbind them. You can begin to diminish the *Fear-Reactivity* that prevents you from accessing unlimited strength, health and performance. You CAN! But you must first realize that your pain, aches, and trauma COMPETE for your ability to transcend the limitation of your self.

Remember that *Fear-Reactivity* is a "tolerance to pain, aches, and trauma." Sustained repetition of any event produces an adaptation. That "progress," that "addiction tolerance," is the *Fear-Reactivity*, which influences your *Self-Image*. The negative feelings and internal dialogue that result attempt to sabotage your freedom, whispering in your ear, telling you how much it hurts, how much better it would be to stop, how much easier it would be to never start.

Pain bites. But its just information. Remember that there is a difference between NOISE and SIGNAL. The noise is all those knotted muscles, weakened tendons and ligaments, dry joint capsules straining under the effort of your movement, your New Beginning. An injury is different. An injury sends an urgent distress signal. You need to learn the difference between the noise of pain and the signal of injury. Through *Body-Flow*, you'll be provided with "biofeedback" which will help you tune out the noise, and amplify the clarity of any signals that you transmit.

And it all begins with proper training. I'll provide you with the chisel and file to truly bring out the details of the Masterpiece which is YOU with my specialized drills which I coined as *Biomechanical Exercise* in the next chapter.

THE DOMINANCE OF VISION

Without **Body-Flow**, you tend to use your vision (and your vestibular system) as your primary information collector to tell you the location and position of your body in space, gravity, and time. Even when you visually misjudge your bodily position and _despite that your Sixth Sense warns you of the error_, you still tend to obey what your eyes show you, overriding your "gut instinct" in nearly every circumstance.

My _Biomechanical Exercise_ in the next chapter will help you prevent your vision from dominating your Sixth Sense. One useful tool for this is **Sensory Deprivation Training** (SDT).

One way of improving the _Sixth Sense_ is to diminish or block sensory input. SDT can be a valuable tool for enhancing technical skills. It does not disrupt motor activities. Actually, sensory-deprived _Biomechanical Exercise_ increases precision and stability while helping you clearly visualize the actual performance goals of the skill.

Ordinarily, you remain largely unaware of gross inefficiency in your movements. How many people know when they are moving with un-coordination and stiffness? You may suspect it when confronted with the opportunity to learn a new skill, but you don't know it in general. Do you consider yourself graceful, masterful in your motion, move like a panther and breath with total ease brimming with energy? Well, you should! It's your birthright to do so! SDT helps you correct your errors by increasing the accuracy and sophistication of your _Mental Blueprint_.

Turn the radio off and find solitude from all other noise. Turn down or switch off the lights or close your eyes (or at least get away from mirrors). Try to reduce all distractions from your practice – a reason that I often refer to this training as _Moving Meditation_.

Fully experience each and every performance goal in the exercise: the angle of your joints, the amplitude of the motion, meshing your exhalation with compression and your inhalation with expansion.

"Strobe" your practice, one repetition sensory deprived, the next not. You will notice enhanced motor sensitivity preserved throughout this drill even when you have full senses operating. Start slowly and carefully and allow your confidence to build.

Having mastered an exercise, you can induce sensory stress with bright flashing lights (as if at a competition) and loud music (as if from the din of the crowding spectators), while on challenging terrain such as wood or concrete, on the grass, on the sand, on pebbles, in the water, barefoot. Each stressful addition or increment (called _Combat Multipliers_ in military psychological training and _Emotional Threshold Training_ in sport psychology) increases the attention required.

This is a very valuable tool because if you remove one channel (your vision), you decrease the noise and increase the signal of the channel you want to amplify – your Sixth Sense!

QUIET AS PROTOCOL

Silence, in most cases, demonstrates efficiency. Have you ever startled someone because of "accidentally" approaching them while in stealth mode? Have you ever watched someone sneak up on someone else? Have you ever watched a cat stalk a bird?

Each muscle poised using the PRECISE amount of force necessary to accomplish the task. This is the actual definition of efficiency:

$$\frac{\text{Useful work}}{\text{Total work}}$$

How much total effort did it require? How much use did you get out of the total effort you expended? That ratio determines the efficiency of that movement.

My philosophy mentor, Doctor Jonathon Ellsworth Winter, once said, *"Don't speak unless you can improve on the silence."* This noise applies to movement. Move while producing the least amount of noise as you touch the ground and you demonstrate masterful muscle control. *"Silence speaks to me secretly, everything,"* Dr. Winter also said. If you want to know the degree of your coordination, agility, and balance, listen rather than watch. The less you hear, the greater the skill level.

WHAT IS THE MOST CRITICAL ASPECT OF SIXTH SENSE?

Mechanoreception is the most critical aspect of *Sixth Sense* in that it tells you where you are, what you are doing, what is being done to you. It programs your implicit memory, so that you remember how to do things as simple as tying your shoes. It is the bag from which your intuition feeds, from whence your "gut instinct" derives its information!

It's the key to unlocking the distinction between you and your environment, between the Map and the Landscape. *Mechanoreception* senses what occurs within you as well as sensing the events in your environment and comprises a blending of Position, Movement and Tension sense.

This information must be specifically manicured to unleash **Body-Flow** however. Remember that internal model which represents you in your environment three-dimensionally in your brain, from moment-to-moment? Your *Mental Blueprint*? Now, remember how you read earlier that your *Mental Blueprint* is the physical aspect of your *Self-Image*?

All right, when do you receive mechanoreceptive information along the path from Spine to Brain Stem to Cerebral Cortex? You receive mechanoreceptive information FIRST don't you? You receive before your thoughts, before your vision, before your vestibular system's info. So, what does that tell you?

It tells you that influencing your *Mental Blueprint* gives you the earliest opportunity to unbinding your flow! It tells you that FEEDING your mechanoreceptors deliberately <u>PROGRAMS your</u> *Mental Blueprint*. Doing so systematically changes your *Self-Image* - vanquishes that little mind-kill of negative internal dialogue, unhinges **Fear-Reactivity**, and unbinds your flow.

Most people really never see the beauty of the world, because they remain locked within the pungent prejudice of a *Mental Blueprint* dictated by **Fear-Reactivity**, and a *Self-Image* manufactured from *Bound-Flow*. Once you access your *Sixth Sense*, you will be able to fully control your motions. Some call it grace, poise, or fluidity – they all refer to **Body-Flow**.

It's really the difference between Being and Becoming, between being your natural powerful inheritance, and becoming your Patterns of **Fear-Reactivity** and identifying with 'it' as your Self-Image. It involves the difference between spontaneously and creatively responding to your internal and external environment, and reacting to the world in knee-jerk fashion.

I have one client worth over $50 million dollars and he dwells in utter anguish, his armor so thick and so burdensome that he ripples with injury, with decay, and with an ego so dominant that he doesn't know how to leverage it out. He's Become so much, but finds no peace in the laborious administration of what only he can direct for fear of "losing" all he "built up around" him-Self. He doesn't know how to "just be" himself. He doesn't know who that is.

Another client of mine, a famous celebrity, worked hard her entire life to Become Big. But she didn't realize the difference, didn't know how to stay the path of Being herself and Becoming a star. Now, people identify her with her characters, with the glitz and glamour, with the sensationalism and the intrigue. She feels like a slave to her expectations of her career and the public's expectations of her life.

A big name trainer in the fitness industry requested my guidance many years ago. We've been in constant contact since then, because he wanted to Become a Big-Name, but didn't know how. I cautioned him that he needed to just Be himself and share his unique genius and talents with people genuinely and the abundance would necessarily follow. He walks the line each day fearing his inability to Become his dreams; not recognizing that what lay underneath those fears is something greater, more fulfilling and more rewarding than anything he could imagine.

All of these people have something in common. They lack a fully realized *Mental Blueprint*. They assumed shape (external appearance or external validation) provides happiness, but shape follows FORM. Form is your integrity – what is integral to BEING you. Only Form can unbind your flow. Shape can only react in the way it was conditioned. Form can adapt, create an appropriate, efficient shape for every situation.

Through my training in **Body-Flow**, all of them, like thousands of others, have become successful at Being true to integrity and achieve greater success than they thought possible. They achieved this through clearing the channel to the most fundamental information in human life: their ability to move, breath and structure themselves in a three dimensional world.

There's a groove. There's a sweet spot in every moment where your breath, your movements, and your alignment all seem to coalesce into a perfect symphony. We've all experienced it at one time or another in our lives. And it wasn't a chemical High. It wasn't a cheap thrill. It certainly wasn't the fulfillment of some expectation – because we know how anti-climatic that is.

It was about the harmony, the synergy, and the flow of the moment. How everything fit together and created something greater than the sum of the parts, in such a way that it was the perfect blend.

It all begins with truly BEING part of the environment, of losing the distinction between you and it.

In martial arts, the pseudo-masterful, the pigeons wearing eagle's feathers, present this as some esoteric component to fighting with such whack-job inaccessibility that no one believes them capable of it without decades of skill refinement. Hogwash and horse-puckey!

MASTERY IS ALWAYS AND ALREADY YOURS!

There's nothing inaccessible about Being truly an inextricably intertwined aspect of the world. It's done every moment in surfing, in dancing, in hiking, in playing with your children at the beach, in negotiating and debating, in community service, in any activity whatsoever!

It all begins with how you feed your *Mental Blueprint*. And *Mechanoreception* is the doorway to that hunger.

You are the architect of your own mastery. You can construct a building using **Fear-Reactivity** with walls so thick no one can harm you, though the inhabitants will eventually die of starvation (perhaps even cannibalization.) Or you can compose a sculpture moment-to-moment to free your creativity, your improvisation, your innovation.

I've been working with people for nearly a decade with the information contained in **Body-Flow**. It's worked for thousand and thousand of clients around the world from every walk of life, for every challenge faced.

How do I specifically unlock my potential? Form.

In the early stages of learning an exercise, you use your voluntary nervous system to assist in integrating the huge amount of information from mechanoreception. Eventually you will be able to rely almost entirely on automatic processes to manage the tasks. However, you must systematically feed mechanoreception the position, movement and tension.

If you struggle and strain, attempt to fight through, overpower, brace against, resist or short cut the exercise, you condition those little reactions. I see this time and time again – more bad habits learned than anything else in an exercise. Exercise wasn't even meant to learn good habits, but rather to feel the sweet spot, get your groove, find the zone.

What I'm teaching you will prevent you from recruiting muscles that serve no purpose in controlling those movements. Have you ever watched someone throw a ball for the first time in later life, not as a child, but as an adult? Or maybe swing a tennis racket, or jump on a snowboard, or... compete in a fighting sport? They move like bricks with shoes, grimacing like twisted metal under the strain of TOO MUCH TENSION!

Tension in muscles that are supposed to be relaxed may well be a cause of MOST injuries. Learning FORM is therefore essential, not only for efficiency, but also for preventing injury. Neglect of this basic rule is commonplace among many who strain inefficiently, using brute force to perform skills that could be performed effortlessly by getting out of their own way, but unbinding all of that superfluous tension.

HOW DO I TURN KNOW-ANCES INTO NEW-ANCES? DO EVERYTHING FOR THE FIRST TIME.

In light of the information you take in, if you view your exercise, or if you view life in general as one endless cycle of repetition, how do you hope to learn anything new? How do you hope to improve?

This is one of the greatest detriments brought on by the "fitness industry" – addiction to SET/REP SCHEMES. By absolute ascription to quantifying movement, nuance disappears, precision deteriorates, and boredom lets loose its gremlin to wreak havoc within your performance, health and strength.

So often we hear the cliché of keeping the "Beginner's Mind." And this elusive concept becomes quickly lost on us. How can we look at something we've done before with an inner dialogue that tells us there's nothing new about that which we're doing?

Well, therein lay the answer to the puzzle. You can't look at that which you prejudice as "known." This is one of the reasons that *Biomechanical Exercise* is critical to reclaiming your **Body-Flow** – the exercise selection is sophisticated. No matter how long you've been doing them, there will always be room for improvement. There will always be a recalibration of your performance goals: one time a component lacks efficiency with breathing, another time with efficient structure, another time with efficient movement… then another component, then another, then the transition.

By approaching *Biomechanical Exercise* from the perspective that every time you do something it's for the first time, you gain access to a clear signal and shut out all of the noise which boredom, that cancerous prejudice of the inner dialogue, creates. Boredom and prejudice diminish your sensory-information gathering; make you dull and lackluster, learning little, and promoting stagnation.

Instead of ignoring what you consider KNOW-ances and going for repetition, scrutinizing your exercise for NEW-ances. The wonderment, fun, exhilaration infects your every movement. It excites your nervous system rewarding you with access to your natural talent, genius and abundance.

Most importantly, by approaching your training as practice (as viewing each movement as 'new'), you sophisticate your movement capabilities, and as a result, diminish your negative inner dialogue… and eventually cease it.

This could probably be one of the most important transferred aspects of **Body-Flow**: the ability to view life like your exercise - as one fabulous Journey of discovery!

WHAT ARE THE THIRTEEN ESSENTIAL ELEMENTS OF BODY-FLOW?

I have taught you four of the elements to **Body-Flow**:

- ***Fear-Reactivity*** dis-integrates Breathing, Structure and Movement; re-integrate them to reclaim **Body-Flow**
- Respond to the Signal - don't React to the Noise
- Be Efficiently Effective
- Do Everything for the First Time

The next nine elements to **Body-Flow** are:

- Balance Tension and Relaxation
- Find Stability through Mobility
- Suspend the Concept of Technique
- Melt into the Composition of Forces
- Activate your Core through Being Breathed BY Performance
- Reveal Perpetual Exercise
- The Ending Determines the Beginning
- Make your Whole Greater than the Sum of your Parts
- Move from Recovery to Coordination to Refinement

How do I move from Tension to Relaxation? Tonus.

A very useful phenomenon is muscle tone, or *tonus*. **Tonus** is defined as <u>the residual tension of a muscle when at rest</u>. Remember, *Residual Muscle Tension*? Okay, good. Now, hold that on the back burner for a moment.

Rest is defined as the condition in which all interacting forces are at equilibrium and no measurable work is performed.

Muscle tone is a neurally induced persistent condition which varies greatly from person to person. Tone varies so greatly because it's mostly a function of the amount of work you subject your muscles to.

On one extreme, overworked and overdeveloped muscles produce *hyper-tonicity*, a condition best described as "muscle-boundness" – *Bound-Flow*, permanent Patterns of **Fear-Reactivity**. It is this "tension" or chronic muscle contraction that you seek to remove.

On the other extreme, deconditioned, underdeveloped muscles exhibit hypo-tonicity, or "flabbiness." Both extremes inhibit smooth and efficient movement.

Muscle tension is not bad in and of itself. Without it, you would crumple to the floor like a sack of guts. Tension keeps you animate. However, as I began, you have two specific villains burglarizing your health, strength and performance: *Residual Muscle Tension* and *Sensory Motor Amnesia*.

Relaxation is not good in and of itself. If you are too relaxed, joints destabilize, organs move into hazardous positions, you cannot operate your lungs, and a whole host of evil little flaccid events. Tension is necessary for daily living, and essential for the realization of your natural talent, genius and abundance.

It's your excess tension that concerns me. It needs to be in balance. I don't think too many of you need to worry about being too relaxed, right? Not in America, anyway, that's for sure.

Tonus in a muscle is comparable to the idling of an engine. A well-tuned engine idles smoothly and responds swiftly when called on to work. The engine that idles too fast is inherently wasteful. The engine that idles poorly sputters and stalls. Good tonus, like the smoothly idling muscle engine, enhances the smooth initiation and work performance whenever it is needed. The "ignition" is never turned off.

Tension and relaxation are two wheels of the same cart. You cannot get anywhere without both. In order to generate maximal tension, you must have maximal relaxation. Therefore, you must ensure that your muscle tone is both necessary and sufficient: *necessary* in that no more tonus than you need, and *sufficient* in that you are able to be called upon for the activities of your life.

When you encounter points of excess tension, or tension which hinders a movement, breathe into and melt the EXCESSIVE tone in those muscles. Have enough to accomplish the task and no more than necessary. This is the essence of efficiency. Produce the most amount of useful work from the least amount of total work.

Find Stability through Mobility: Zero Position & Zeno's Paradox, The Concept of Technique is Absent, and Composition of Forces

All movement balances stability and mobility. Every movement you make both stabilizes your joints and moves the bones like levers.   But there are two sets of forces acting upon you, from within and from without. Let's look at those for a moment:

Internally, what creates your internal movement? You move when your nerves direct your muscles to work. These impulses cause muscles to pull your bones. Your muscles and bones attached by tendons cause motion around your joints.

Externally, your body is always subject to forces that can cause it to shift position or remain stable, to accelerate or decelerate. In everyday life you are usually unaware of the forces acting on you, but as soon as you begin a new movement, these forces become part of your conscious awareness.

The most constant force is gravity, which exerts a pull that keeps you rooted to Earth. The point at which your body is in contact with the ground or with some other object, such as an opponent in martial arts, is the point at which two other forces come into play: friction and reaction.

Friction is the resistance that a moving object encounters when it comes into contact with the surface of another object.

Reaction is the term taken from Newton's law, which states that for every action there is an equal and opposite reaction.

Finally, motion slows by drag, a function of acceleration through the flow of air, which opposes your forward momentum.

The relative strength of these forces varies, depending on the activity and the speed of your movement. Gravity, Friction, Drag and Reaction account for the external forces which you encounter. Of course, as I wrote above there's also the internal forces – the balance of tension and relaxation. You need to do more than balance all of these forces. You must equalize them.

Imagine yourself as a top lying on its side. Its function remains hidden because gravity dominates it. Spin the top somewhat. Drag and friction cause a beastly display of movement, and gravity of course yanks the top back down to its side after only a few revolutions. Spin it perfectly but into another object and the reaction knocks over the top. Of course, in a vacuum, with a perfectly flat environment containing no obstacles and no gravity, the top would remain spinning forever. The top will have achieved – **Zero Position**: the state where all forces acting upon an object equalize. It is that delicate stability achieved when all forces cancel each other out equaling ZERO.

The top perfectly displays **Zero Position** in its spinning even when not in a vacuum. Once spun, and without interference from external obstacles, it "Breaks Gravity" achieving the temporary state of perfect equilibrium.

Notice that lying on its side does not equal **Zero Position** for the top. The top serves no function, has not expressed its essence, just lumped on the floor like a doorstop. How many of you live your lives like this? I know I did for too long.

Zero Position is a constant juggling battle of feeling the synergy of all of the forces internal and external, of experiencing the harmony of equalizing – finding the perfect blend of them – and getting out of the way of the *Design* of the top to reveal the synchronously flow.

However, you don't live in a vacuum, and you always have external forces acting upon you, causing friction, dragging you, weighing you down and eliciting reactions within you. You don't have one mere point of balance, because you are jointed. You constantly experience a network of ineffective and inefficient tensions throughout. You continually have outside forces prodding, poking, punching at you.

Don't view **Body-Flow** as a series of connection stances. Stance is something you move THROUGH! It's a snapshot in time. Imagine looking at an old movie reel. Each frame appears to be still, captured in a prison of stances. What you rob the reel of is motion. It is a MOTION picture after all, and the spinning of the reel gives life to the inanimation of stance. You cannot disassemble motion into frames of positions, nor can you take a collection of stances and create motion without the critical ingredient of transitional MOTION!

This is explained in a very old Greek logic puzzle called *Zeno's Paradox*. It goes like this: take an arrow and shoot it towards a bull's eye 10 yards away. Now in order for that arrow to travel to the target, it must reach half way. And in order for it to reach half way, it must travel one half of that half. Of course to travel one half of one half, it must again, travel half of that distance, and so on ad infinitum. The paradox is that in order for anything to travel a distance it must go half of the distance, and there is an infinite digression of halves. The result, it's impossible for anything to ever travel anywhere!

So what's the solution to the paradox? MOTION, of course! What those snapshots in time rob from logical scrutiny is that the arrow is NEVER at ANY one of those points. It is always traveling THROUGH those points.

What's the moral of the story? Never view **Body-Flow** as a collection of points, snapshots, stances. **Body-Flow** is always moving THROUGH positions that efficiently integrate breathing, structure and MOVEMENT!

Solving *Zeno's Paradox* and finding **Zero Position** in your life can only be achieved by staying in motion. *"Contrary to popular belief, the novice must be taught from a base of mobility to progress to stability,"* write Dr. Verkhoshanky and Dr. Siff in *Supertraining*. You'll never find your groove, if you're on the floor like the doorstop top. You need to spin. You need to fly. You need to experience failure and bounce on to the next course. You need to get hit and absorb the blow while rapidly recovering your **Zero Position**. You need to stay in motion in order to find that peace in the storm.

I know it's something that I could only live through the tumultuous fury of fighting. I realize to many that fighting seems anything but peaceful. However there's something beautiful in a fight, something pure in it. In it, if you can remain calm, and do that which is necessary and sufficient: not hyper-tense – not hypo-tense, and if in that storm you find the Eye, you've blended with the event. It becomes one frighteningly elegant display of truth – **Zero Position**.

For me fighting was never about the winning and the losing, but rather canceling out all of the forces, including myself – actively creating zero. It was a strategy initially for defeating opponents. By creating zero, by focusing not on winning or losing but on canceling out any attempts at unbalancing "us" my opponents quickly would become frustrated. Their frustration led to over-tense attempts, and that EXCESS TENSION caused their demise each and every time. I "watched" countless opponents fall this way, fall due to their own undoing, unbalancing themselves through their own internal dissonance.

But after years of years of fighting in world caliber events internationally, I came to appreciate **Zero Position** in and of itself. I came to just love to "Be" in that moment. It's hard to describe, but any truly competitive athlete understands. The word "competition" itself derives from the Latin root of the words *con* and *petire*, which mean "to seek together." No political diplomacy ever equaled what has been done through sport. Athletes from every nation have an intuitive connection to each other – a mutual respect for that collective "seeking together" of that *Zero horizon*.

For you philosophy buffs, you may know that Hegel coined the concept:

Thesis => Antithesis => Synthesis

However, what some of you may not know is that he actually creatively "adopted" this concept from Fichte, who originally named it:

Position => Opposition => Composition

During my fighting career, it was Fichte's concept which I creatively adopted as a combative strategy. You see, what makes martial arts problematic is that they are a collection of techniques. Technique is some lunatic marketing innovation created by entrepreneurs to deceive the masses into believing they can fight. But techniques are as ineffable and useless as Plato's ideal forms.

Many people in many places have read my outright criticism of martial arts – calling their educational format a farce. It's an interesting crowd to enrage because they love to puff and pound their chest, and yet when it's "go time" the doubt of the efficacy of their beloved "techniques" creeps stealthily into their heads. I encapsulated this understanding by saying:

The concept of technique is absent.

Confidence in a technique is not confidence in yourself. I'll explain why. Every technique or stance is a Position. To every position, there is an opposite technique which counters that initial technique. In other words, to every Position, there is Opposition. By their very nature these techniques and stances create resistance. To every physical thesis, there is an antithesis. The right and the wrong, the good and the evil... everything cut into this tiny perfect little black and white Bizzaro world.

So what's the solution to the dualistic schism? Well, you should be able to figure it out by now. What's **Zero Position**? How do you solve *Zeno's Paradox*?

Composition of Forces. This is why everywhere you read me guiding you to find a melody of your movement (*Flow*), a chorus of your resources (*Synergy*), and a symphony of your life (*Harmony*).

A Position is something you only PASS THROUGH. You are never AT any point, but merely a visitor on your merry way of **Body-Flow**. You cannot take an flowing experience and break it down into a sequence of fixed stances and techniques. What worked one moment was only relevant to that moment. As Miyamoto Musashi, arguably the greatest swordsmen of all time wrote, *"you can see the SHAPE by which I am victorious, but what remains invisible to you is the form by which I guarantee victory."* Form: the underlying mechanics which permit flow – the efficient integration of movement, breathing and structure.

In fighting, finding a **Composition of Forces** consistently provided me and all of the fighters who I have trained maximum success with minimal energy expenditure. Blending, folding, melding, joining the tumultuous chaos of the engagement brings about a certain objective beauty.

But how many of you can get out of the way of opposition? How many of you feel like you have these granite walls to protect? What do you face in your life, from one moment to the next which feels like one collision after another?

It's **Fear-Reactivity** which causes you to adopt a position, which gives you the impression you are beset by raging opposition from every quarter. But it's all an illusion which you dispel once you reclaim your natural **Body-Flow**.

You can find a harmony with the forces which assault those sad, immobile souls who because of ego, because of the little troglodyte called by **Fear-Reactivity** remain locked in an eternal struggle within themselves as well as with others. However, by unbinding your flow, by removing your **Fear-Reactivity**, you compose these forces into a tapestry of health, strength and performance.

Some call it Grace, others Poise. Many call it Composure as in the ability to compose. For me, it's the amalgam experience of Synergy, Flow and Harmony.

..

WHAT IS THE GOAL OF BIOMECHANICAL EXERCISE™?
INTEGRATION.

Quite simply, the goal of *Biomechanical Exercise* is to efficiently integrate your Breathing, Movement and Structure, and to make seamless the transition of one motion to the next.

Physical activity of any kind depends primarily on neuromuscular mechanisms: special sensors in the muscles, tendons, and joints that detect position, velocity, and tension; special sensors in the hands, feet, and skin that detect vibration, pain, and pressure; and the vestibular apparatus near your inner ear that acts as your inertial guidance for postural equilibrium. These sensors stabilize, assess, and direct the body in time and space. Your bodily awareness owns critical importance for movement mastery and self-image. Acquisition of effective and efficient movement strategies is essential for unlocking your unlimited health, strength and performance.

Biomechanical Exercise is a physical method of what movement scientists call *Functional Neuromuscular Conditioning.* "FNC may be seen to embrace all-around development of function and structure. FNC should be regarded as an entire conditioning system capable of developing any desired type of musculoskeletal fitness." (Siff, _Supertraining,_ p 407.)

Biomechanical Exercise enhances the response of these neuromuscular mechanisms by imposing specific agility, coordination, and balance demands. *Biomechanical Exercise* has a dominant role in all aspects of physical culture, including functioning as rehabilitative and preventative health measures. *Biomechanical Exercise* specifically manufactures Biomechanical Efficiency, which relates to the leverage characteristics of the body, the relative strengths of the different muscle groups controlling the movement of each limb, and the neuromuscular efficiency that orchestrates all movement patterns of the body. [*Neuromuscular Efficiency* relates to how efficiently and intensively one recruits muscle fibers in the appropriate muscle groups to produce the movement pattern accurately and powerfully.]

Unlike the immutable genetic factors that predispose one person to achieve a potential that far exceeds that of another person, both neuromuscular and biomechanical efficiency are profoundly influenced by training and offer a vehicle for producing great increases.

The goal of *Biomechanical Exercise* is to unbind your flow. Though much of the complex physiological activity necessary for movement occurs unconsciously, all human movement requires a coordinated sequence of muscle contractions, changes in various joint positions, and a variation in the tension applied to tendons and ligaments. Becoming aware of the basics in these movement characteristics is the first step to accessing to your unique talent, genius and abundance.

WHAT'S THE DIFFERENCE BETWEEN BODYWEIGHT AND BIOMECHANICAL EXERCISE™?

Bodyweight exercise (BWE), historically known as calisthenics, emphasizes strength, endurance, and flexibility. Calisthenics use the weight of the body to condition the body. Bodyweight exercises must have technical simplicity so that athletes may immediately execute the skill.

Biomechanical Exercise, historically known as acrobatics, emphasizes agility, coordination, and balance. *Biomechanical Exercise* must have technical sophistication so that you may sufficiently unlock your **Body-Flow**.

Biomechanical Exercise once mastered, can be used as bodyweight exercise (for volume, intensity and density), but the reverse is not true. This is because <u>bodyweight exercise lacks the sophistication necessary to unbind your flow</u>.

One way to distinguish the two is to regard *Biomechanical Exercise* as *practice* and bodyweight exercise as *training*. Practice refers to technical rehearsal for recovering, developing, and refining a skill. Training refers to repetition for increasing attributes. Bodyweight exercise movements are so basic that little practice is required. As a result they can be used immediately for training. After conditioning, they may be used for competition against others to demonstrate strength, endurance and flexibility.

Competition can be understood simply as *challenging resistance*. Resistance can be an external opponent, such as an opposing player in a sport or an enemy on the battlefield. Resistance can be understood as an internal opponent, such as resisting muscles, fear of awkward movement, or fear of injury.

It is easier to compete using bodyweight exercise because the standards are quantifiable. However, the grace and poise of *Biomechanical Exercise* is not so easy, because the factors of agility, coordination and balance apply equally to strength, endurance and flexibility. Think of BWE as a military conditioning examination and BME as a gymnastics competition. How do you quantify quality of movement?

Biomechanical Exercise augments the <u>quality</u> of your movement by re-integrating your breathing, movement and structure.

ACTIVATE YOUR CORE THROUGH BEING BREATHED BY PERFORMANCE

Critical to **Body-Flow** is your "core." There's a great deal of conjecture about what constitutes "core." Suffice it to say that your core determines the success, health and strength of your performance in all things. However, let's only address for now just the abdominals.

Body-Flow necessarily involves movement in the three-dimensional world and as a result, the rotational and angular/diagonal properties of muscle action. The stability of your trunk therefore can be found only through improvement of your awareness and attention to core mobility.

You can find many more examples in **Body-Flow**. You can refer to my _Be Breathed_, _Warrior Wellness_, _Grapplers Toolbox_ and _Zdorovye Fitness System_ video courses. They all take the Janda sit-up beyond high-gear and to a level of sophistication not seen anywhere else (and probably it will stay that way for a long time, since everyone in the "industry" focuses on mundane KISS exercises.)

Your abdominal muscles involve both internal and the external portions. The _rectus abdominus_ (your 6-pack) and the _external obliques_. If you get horizontal on the floor for my exercises, you can feel the rectus abdominus flex the spinal column forward 30 degrees. If you move beyond this, you're actually engaging the hip-flexors and going beyond the nature of _Core Activation_.

Your trunk rotates primarily under the power of the external obliques, which definitely get blasted by any type of my exercises. For our purposes here however your focus lay with the Inner Unit: the _transversus abdominus_ and the _lumbar multifidus_. These muscles exist underneath the external abdominals and involve the control of your respiration and your structural core alignment. Furthermore, they contribute to your total health, performance and strength. It's because of your Inner Unit, that you'll hear me eschewing the use of crutches like lifting belts, which inhibit the inner breathing patterns that you need for true strength and performance.

Recent research goes more deeply into understanding this, but to keep it in simple terminology, your Inner Unit must fire slightly before your Outer Unit. If you train only your Outer Unit, as the fitness trends would have you do (well, as most strength and conditioning pundits would have you do), you are rewiring the firing sequence of your _Core Activation_.

It's really too monumental to explain in one book. If you train your Inner Unit to misfire you not only diminish your _Core Activation_, you create structural imbalances that will lead to injury.

How many avid lifters and fitness enthusiasts do you know that after a session suffer massive back spasms (for "no apparent reason") or "throw out their back" from putting on their pants or going to the toilet? The reason of course involves poor, ineffective and misfired _Core Activation_.

My exercise selection will help you address this aspect of _Body-Flow_, and more importantly become aware of it in all exercises and eventually in ALL MOVEMENT IN GENERAL!

Don't misunderstand my emphasis on attention to the Inner Unit as a "targeting" of Inner Unit exercise. It's about training in a way that not only does not interfere with the effective "firing sequence" of your musculature, but also the positive health and performance impact it has if we augment this procedure deliberately through practice.

It's really one of the most important points I can communicate to you. This is HOW you integrate your breathing, movement and alignment. No, this is not the "key" element. It is only one example of one element in integrating all three in one situation. It's far more sophisticated and total bodily than just this one issue. But it's here at this issue that I can illustrate the crux of the matter:

If the Inner Unit impacts breathing and structural alignment, and we interrupt or rewire the firing sequence through any type of training, we adversely impact the total performing organism – YOU!

Contrarily, if we take the natural firing sequence and augment it, you powerfully integrate your breathing, movement and structure in all your activities all the time! This is the key to _Perpetual Exercise_ philosophy and the precursor to understanding **Performance Breathing**.

Read the above carefully. Proper _Core Activation_ is what you always and already have. It's a latent prowess that is your birthright. Certain training methods, especially vogue right now, CREATE FEAR-REACTIVITY by building up the rock-hard armor, specifically conditioning you to insensitivity.

PERPETUAL EXERCISE: EVERY MOMENT IS AN ACT OF CONDITIONING

My breathing techniques receive the most amount of interest it seems, most likely since breathing appears to be the most neglected (hence, the popular breath holding habit) and most impacting element upon strength, health and performance. However, it seems that breathing also has become the most over-engineered aspect exercise, a sad fact that acts to confuse and limit your access to **Body-Flow**.

I hold no interest whatsoever in debating with proponents of other techniques. Researchers present information on both sides. My techniques work for multitudes of athletes, world champions, national coaches, psychologists, physicians, and the average fitness enthusiast alike. I'll present you with some scientific highlights, but let's not stray away from the fact that these are "natural" breathing methods that facilitate and augment your natural talent, genius and performance.

Let's explore some of the common issues you face while breathing.

Oxygen Debt: unlike other bodily cells, muscle cells are uniquely tolerant for temporary oxygen deprivation: a safety factor that enables you to address emergency situations. When activity is increased in intensity or duration to the extent that more oxygen is needed than available, energy is liberated by anaerobic ("without oxygen") chemical processes in the muscles, and you incur an *oxygen debt*.

You can only tolerate the waste products of anaerobic processes (primarily lactic acid) to a certain degree before your muscles can no longer contract. At that point you're exhausted. After you incur an oxygen debt you need a period of mild activity or rest. During that time oxygen consumption will occur at an increased rate until the oxygen debt has been paid and a normal chemical balance of the muscles has been reestablished. Basically, you're heaving, trying to catch up with the exertion. The time you need to recover depends on the magnitude of your debt and of course your level of physical (anaerobic) conditioning.

Your heart and the brain, however, <u>cannot</u> tolerate an oxygen debt. They depend entirely on oxidative energy, and their function suffers immediately when their supply of oxygen falls. Exercise does not affect the oxygen supply of the brain as it does in the heart, where there may be a tremendous increase in the need for oxygen during exercise. This oxygen must be supplied by the coronary circulation. The ability to meet this need of the heart for oxygen is one of the most important factors limiting the intensity and duration of activity.

The method I teach you below, **Performance Breathing**, will help you RECOVER more rapidly from Oxygen Debt than any other technique in existence. Furthermore, it will help you process oxygen at a cellular level more efficiently to supply any needs of your heart and brain.

Breathlessness indicates a degree of oxygen debt that your muscles have incurred through strenuous activity. Of course, your recovery time here is as I described above. How fast you pay back your debt depends upon your breathing method, which is probably insufficient even at rest. Most people cannot access the three levels of breathing, taught in *Performance Breathing*: Clavicular, Intercostal, and Diaphragmatic. Depending upon how poor your muscular habits of breathing are, you increase the degree and recovery period from breathlessness brought about by strenuous activity.

Circulo-Respiratory Distress Pre-2nd Wind: Consider 2nd *Wind* from a neurological standpoint as a possible analogy. It represents an adjustment in the circulo-respiratory process. The adjustment enables you to continue strenuous or prolonged physical activity with renewed vigor and greater comfort.

Preceding the onset of 2nd *Wind*, you experience great physical distress - such as rapid, shallow breathing, an abnormal pulse, and other symptoms of physical distress. You may experience 2nd *Wind* with dramatic suddenness, or may occur so subtly that it goes unnoticed until upon you and the little mind-gremlins return to implore you to stop the strenuous activity.

Respiratory specialists still cannot explain 2nd *Wind*. Since your physical limitation in activity is determined by the circulatory rather than the respiratory system, 2nd *Wind* could be primarily a circulatory adjustment in the midst of strenuous or prolonged activity to meet the oxygen needs in your muscles.

Some neurologists surmise that the cerebrum produces 2nd *Wind* by concentrating on the movement, and as a result facilitates a more efficient neuromuscular coordination. Although their explanations are inadequate, 2nd *Wind* can be described as a sub-cortical response to the needs of working muscles and to concentration on a specific goal. It is entirely possible that the distress you are experiencing is a threshold to a neuromuscular adjustment to the activity.

2nd *Wind* may be a limiting nickname as is. I believe a more accurate description is Gear. There are as many Gears as you have thresholds. For prolonged activity, on one ultra-distance marathon, I crested 40 miles in 4th Gear. 1st Gear of course is your comfort zone. 2nd Gear is your first level of physical distress. It's the point you achieve when you've actually tweaked the metabolic state above "rest." In prolonged running, for most people this is 1-2 miles. People fight it. They associate the distress with their conditioning level... and they quit. They quit when they are only a few steps away from a neurological adaptation. It's a beautiful thing.

Because you're probably associating the physical distress and the phantom aches as your level of conditioning, you 'feel' that you cannot go further. This is why so many coaches preach the "mind over matter" non-sense. That's definitely backwards thinking. It's the MIND that is limited, not the body.

In sport psychology, we call your threshold – toughness. If you push through distress, you create that neurological adaptation (on that day, or event) and you become one increment tougher. With each membrane of mental resistance you puncture, you increase what we call "Mental Toughness." Notice it's not physical toughness. You MENTAL toughness increases by allowing your body to overcome resistance and adapt to it.

It's Matter over Mind. It's your Mind, your dirty little demons that tries to convince you to stop, that you're not in good enough condition, that you're not young enough, strong enough... And it's all an illusion. It's all chemicals talking in your head.

Performance Breathing carries you through the physical distress, and will as a result increase your mental toughness – how much you can take before you quit. There's no other breathing method in the world that addresses this in the midst of exerting effort. You can't sit down and relax. You are in the middle of some crisis, or some important event, a sport, a negotiation, an attack… The urgency requires you to perform. Only ***Performance Breathing*** addresses this.

Breath Holding: It is never advisable to hold the breath during any movement even though this seems to be a natural phenomenon during "exercises of effort." Holding the breath closes the epiglottis and increases the intra-thoracic pressure, compresses the large veins of the thorax, and interferes with the return of blood to the heart, and increases the intra-cerebral pressure, which may lead to aneurysm, as well as migraine and burst capillaries in the face. It is important on any movement that the epiglottis is not closed.

Hypoxic versus Hypercapnic: Near the close of the 19th Century, Russian Physiologist Verigo and Dutch Scientist Bohr independently discovered that without CO_2, oxygen remains bound to hemoglobin, unreleased and incapable of being utilized by our tissues. As a result there is an oxygen deficiency in tissues such as our brain, kidneys and heart, as well as a significant increase in our blood pressure.

Russian and former Soviet research, by men like Dr. V. Frolov, Dr. K. Buteyko and Prof. R. Strelkov (Frolov, *Endogenous Breathing*) surmised that deep breathing serves as the root cause of many illnesses. Deep-breathers suffer from O2 starvation and so they "over-breathe" which begins the cycle called the *Hyperventilation Feedback Loop*.

Over-Breathing: Notice how a person holding his breath becomes increasingly hyperactive. Over time the level of CO_2 increases dramatically causing the rapid consumption of O2. This hyperactivity continues until syncope (unconsciousness) – a method used in martial arts to expedite strangulation techniques. The cause of O2 deficiency is not due to the lack of O2 presence, but by the lack of CO_2 retention.

Over-breathing causes O2 deficiency. If we breathe too much, we have less O2 in our body. Two methods of breathing developed from this understanding: hypoxic (or lowered oxygen count) and hypercapnic (or saturated with carbonic gas) breathing. Dr. Vladimir Frolov (*Endogenous Respiration*) concluded from his research that both methods intend the same goal but achieve it through different means:

"Buteyko achieved positive results raising the concentration of carbonic gas in the lungs. Strelkov, in turn, obtained the identical result by lowering the oxygen content in the lungs. The paradox solves itself if we compare oxygen concentrations in both methods. It turned out that what united them was an approximately identical hypoxia regime (lower oxygen content)."

For general training, the conventional method of breathing entails the *Power Breathing Technique*: This hypoxic method was researched by a Russian scientist Professor R. Strelkov and was propagated by Pavel Tsatsouline in the West. Power increases immediately, but fine and complex motor skills such as in any physical activity suffer.

Urgency demands immediate performance increases, such as with military and law enforcement personnel. Some people choose immediate results over longevity due to the short career window of professional sports.   When you do, you choose to results by shaving a few minutes off the end of your life.

In **Body-Flow** however you reclaim what is always and already yours. The results come (and eventually exceed those of Power pundits). However, to do this, you need to allow your breathing to be produced by your structure and movement. I coined this technique - **Performance Breathing**: A hypercapnic method was researched by Russian scientist Dr. K. Buteyko, and was modified by Alexander Retuinskih, founder of the ROSS Training System and Distinguished Coach of Russia, and expanded through research and implementation by yours truly over the past decade.

Basically, **Performance Breathing** involves two primary points:

On compression, allow an exhale; on expansion, allow an inhale. Notice I wrote "allow" – not create. This is what I mean by calling my one video course on the topic _Be Breathed_. I did not call it _Start Breathing_ nor did I name it _Learn to Breath more effectively_. I didn't even call it _Breath_! Your goal is to be breathed by the motion of your movement and structure. As you bend over, a natural compression forces the air out of your lungs. As you stand back straight, the air naturally sucks back into your lungs as your thoracic cavity opens.

Perform fine motor skills at the end of the exhalation, before inhalation. This is called the _Control Pause_ – the moment when your body is at the most complete rest possible (from a mechanical perspective. Ultimately, the _Control Pause_ also happens in between heart beats.)

Now let me give you an example of how to put this in practice.

Performance Breathing Exercise:

> Lay on your back on the floor.
>
> Relax your entire body.
>
> Exhale forcefully by contracting your entire core while bringing your naval towards your spine.
>
> Tilt your pelvis forward and upward as if rolling up your spine, tense your glutes and abs, and grip your feet into the ground like you preparing to dig in to receive a charge.
>
> Hold for 2 seconds.
>
> Slightly release the tension on your core. Do NOT deliberately inhale! What you should experience is a sucking-in of air. This is due to the release of tension in the muscles around the lungs. The negative back pressure vacuums in the exact amount of air you need.
>
> Now, exhale again with an explosive release, NOT a grunt. To do so, tighten your core even more than your first attempt. Really bear down. Tighten your glutes even more strongly.
>
> Hold for 2 seconds.

Repeat this procedure until you have done a total of ten **Performance Breathing** exhalations. Few abdominal workouts even compare to the effectiveness of this exercise.

Key Points:

Exhalation is active (by *Core Activation*); inhalation is passive (by core relaxation – or deactivation).

Do not create intra-cerebral pressure. No red faces! You should be able to carry on a conversation while using **Performance Breathing**.

No breathing method guarantees safety. Responsibly incorporate all technical points: proper movement nuances, proper structural alignment, and proper breathing. Dr. Vladimir Frolov (*Endogenous Respiration*) writes that, *"Scientists believe the key to understanding what health is lies with longevity. It is said, "the one who lives longest feels better."* YOU decide which method you use. Your body is your God-given gift. Treat it as you would treat your Church. Act responsibly with your health. You are responsible

With **Performance Breathing**, your most skilled goals occur at the end of the exhale. This is when your **Body-Flow** is most in sync with the environment, like an archer shooting an arrow, a painter placing brush to canvas, or a martial artist letting fly a fist. Since activity occurs at the end of an exhalation, you performs with optimal function.

Performance Breathing balances health and performance, which should be your default setting. Unless your life or career is on the line, go with Performance Breathing. You'll feel better, you'll tap into your **Body-Flow**, and eventually you'll exceed in results as well as in age, your breath-holding counter-parts.

Basically, **Performance Breathing** is for, by, and of PERFORMANCE. You cannot be a marksman with Power Breathing, nor an archer, nor an efficient fighter. You can't do Power Breathing and paint, drive your car, negotiate in the board room, fix an engine, catch a ball, ride a wave, or play with your child.

Increasing blood pressure and heart rate, switching blood volume to large muscles (decreasing digital dexterity), significantly diminishes and prohibits accuracy and precision. **Performance Breathing** however, approximates the gains, and through practice exceeds the gains of *Power Breathing*. More importantly not only does Performance Breathing not adversely affect, but it greatly improves performance and health.

I teach numerous different *Techniques* of **Performance Breathing** such as Normalizing, Vibration, Alternating, Punctuated, Flushing, Waving, and Yield-Halt-Overcome. However, for this course on **Body-Flow**, you'll only need the basics of what I provided above.

The final point here is that **Performance Breathing** does not regard targeting your performance in some sport, some vocation, or some recreation. Performance Breathing ultimately is about your performance as a human being. This is HUMAN PERFORMANCE I'm talking about. That's the goal! This is where your strength and health meet.

What is your level of sophistication at being YOU? You should be able to walk into any activity and within days, if not minutes approximate any skill because you have had all this time that you've been mastering the one necessary and sufficient tool you own – you!

Performance Breathing is about exercising perpetually, at every moment in every action – seeking your optimal function, uncovering your ***Body-Flow*** in all things. Understanding this simple statement should have the single most profound impact upon your life.

THE ENDING DETERMINES THE BEGINNING

How do you learn a new exercise? Motor scientists believe that unfamiliar activities are under more of your conscious control than movements that you know well. For example, when you first learn a new skill, such as a martial arts technique, a tennis serve or driving a car, you consciously direct that movement in response to feedback from your senses. Because you are unsure of yourself, you need to watch yourself constantly, checking the position of your arms, legs, and torso, to see that you are executing the skill correctly.

Some researchers conclude that after you become proficient at a movement, your conscious muscle control switches gradually to the cerebellum, the part of the brain concerned especially with the coordination and equilibrium. Researchers believe this non-conscious part of your brain, is better equipped to direct a familiar activity with efficiency and accuracy.

After you have learned a complex sequence of movements, such as a kinetic chain, some studies indicate that simpler actions of your routine become automatic, while more difficult movements still demand conscious attention. Similarly, while performing an activity that demands responses to outside stimuli, such as hitting a baseball or catching a Frisbee, movements that follow a predictable pattern may proceed at an unconscious level. At the same time, sudden changes in your situation, such as being thrown a ball that curves, engage your attention at both conscious and unconscious levels.

As I wrote earlier, your goal is to view everything you do as the first time which you are doing it. This will keep your CNS excited and keep boredom from creeping in. More importantly, it keeps life fresh, mysterious and engaging.

The best way to learn a new skill depends on how easily you can isolate the components of a movement. Learning how to shoot a basketball, for example, is best done by practicing the entire motion. The individual steps of that activity are too closely related to separate them into elements that can be practiced on their own. However, one can still find proper integration of breathing, movement and structure in compressed skills.

On the other hand, studies show that the best way to learn a skill involving steps that are relatively independent of each other is to break the exercise down into simpler fundamentals and practice these components until you can perform them correctly. Research demonstrates that the more meaningful the components, the easier they are to learn.

In other words, as you practice individual skills, you should separate them into segments that are easy to practice, but not so small and insignificant that it becomes difficult to relate to the exercise as a whole. You must be able to keep in mind just how the movement fits into the larger organization of the chain.

In **Body-Flow**, you shall find a selection of *Biomechanical Exercises* All of these exercises are composed of three *Components*: a beginning, a middle and an ending. Each of these components involves the integration of your breathing, movement and structure.

Weaving the ending component of one exercise to the beginning component of another exercise seamless produces a *Kinetic Chain*.

Recap:

Elementary Motor Component: a skill integrating a particular action of movement, structure, and breathing.

Biomechanical Exercise   a skill comprising a series (beginning, middle and ending) of elementary motor components.

Kinetic Chain: a series where the ending component of one Biomechanical Exercise meshes seamlessly with the beginning component of another.

Russian researchers discovered that teaching the segments of a new movement in their sequential order from start to finish is not necessarily as effective as teaching the action in the reverse order (Vorobyev, 1978). They examined the effect of breaking down movements into basic components and having athletes learn each element separately before attempting the whole movement. This method of component learning also proved to be superior to the conventional method of natural sequence learning.

For each *Biomechanical Exercise* there is a BEGINNING, MIDDLE, and an ENDING component. Once you understand the breakdown process of beginning, middle and ending elementary motor components, you gain the ability to engineer the educational sequence of movement:

Forward Engineering: Learning components from beginning to ending

Reverse Engineering: Learning components from ending to beginning

Lateral Engineering: Learning middle components, then beginning and ending

These tools work differently for individual learning styles.

One of the crucial secrets to **Body-Flow** is the *movement-in-between*. Every *Biomechanical Exercise* has beginning, middle and ending elementary motor components. Tie together *Biomechanical Exercise* into *kinetic chains*. Do this by breaking *Biomechanical Exercise* into elementary motor components.

How is this possible? The goal is to discover that the ending component of one *Biomechanical Exercise* flows seamlessly into the beginning component of another *Biomechanical Exercise* forming the chain. Realize that there is no beginning and ending to movement. Rather, movement in life is composed of only middle components. There is only transition! This is one of the most powerful statements in this book!

Realize the movement-in-between and you gain the ability to:

Analyze any movement as sequences of building blocks

Alter and combine building blocks into any sequences

All movement is practice – everything you do is an act of conditioning!

I refer here of course to *Perpetual Exercise*. Life doesn't stop, so why should your exercise? You've always been preparing for a competition – the Game of life. You've always been practicing an instrument – you!

Life is composed of one endless series of middle components. *Biomechanical Exercise* is the micro of the macro. The more that you compose Kinetic Chains, the more creativity you express, the more that you unlock your ability to spontaneously respond optimally to any situation with ease, grace, and poise.

When you reclaim your **Body-Flow** through the *Biomechanical Exercise* I depict in this book, you'll make a most essential discovery. It probably won't mean the same thing on the first read as on your 100th read after hours and hours and hours of practice. This book will always bring you new discoveries, always provide you with new insight to yourself – to your innate talent, genius and abundance. This is the discovery…

You're always and already masterful. Trust me; thousands of people have discovered this through emancipation from **Fear-Reactivity**. They had NO IDEA that underneath such simple bodily habits lay such boundless energy, such amazing creativity and such timeless passion.

All of your life's experiences are not wasted! They are all going to be retranslated by your Central Nervous System. Of that stored information can be rather suddenly transformed into instantly accessible bodily wisdom.

The goal is for you to deepen you daily practice… every day. Go deeper. Get sophisticated! Have fun! Play hard!

It's all up to you, and it's all within your grasp, and it's always been there waiting for you to unbind your flow, and reclaim your unlimited health, strength and performance.

FROM RECOVERY TO COORDINATION TO REFINEMENT

Bruce Lee, applying his study of Taoism to martial art, said that when beginning martial art a punch is just a punch. During study, a punch becomes more than merely a punch. After mastery, a punch becomes just a punch again.

When beginning *Biomechanical Exercise* an exercise will be just an exercise. After you study, practice, and explore *Biomechanical Exercise* an exercise will become more than just an exercise. It will become a sophisticated array of components (beginning, middle, and ending) and elements (breathing, movement and alignment). After significant mastery of *Biomechanical Exercise* an exercise becomes just an interwoven piece of this wellness tapestry that is your **Body-Flow** – it returns again to being just an exercise.

Your development therefore can be represented in three phases: recovery, development, and refinement.

Recovery Phase

Ego – emotions of pride, anger, frustration, embarrassment, and fear – intruded on your ability to see an exercise. Your ego competes for your health, strength and performance. Ego is expressed in an action – in acting out your pride, anger, frustration, embarrassment, and fear.

Egotistical actions produce outcomes to which one adapts. As one adapts, one progresses and becomes capable of executing greater actions of the same.

Learning an exercise is not simple; because to truly learn it, you must suspend your ego, you must unbind your flow, remove your **Fear-Reactivity**. This requires vigorous study, practice, and exploration. As you do, you begin to release your unlimited potential. In this *recovery phase* of your development, you reclaim authority over your natural talent, genius and abundance. In the *recovery phase*, you begin to turn on the lights in the basement of your Self-Image, so that you can begin to clean up the mess your ego has made of your health, strength and performance – the creation of Patterned **Fear-Reactivity**.

Development Phase

As you study, practice and explore, you see the implications of the *Essential Elements of Body-Flow*. Each exercise is a sophisticated composite of principles and concepts, methods and applications. Through your study you gain the crucial ability to differentiate between these characteristics.

An exercise gains qualities and dimensions you did not and could not have known because of the rose-colored glasses ego paints. Now, you can look at yourself and at others and see flaws and perfections in exercise technique. Devoid of ego, you can move forward and restore a strong foundation and sturdy structure to your Mental Blueprint.

Refinement Phase

After mastery of the basics of *Biomechanical Exercise*, you see each component as a piece of a completed puzzle. You can pick up a jigsaw piece and, from its design, know its location and purpose in portraying the total mosaic of your health and strength.

Exercises become refined tools now, as means to an end. You gain the ability to see an exercise within its total context. Whereas in the development phase you gained the discernment to differentiate between principles and concepts, methods and applications, in the Refinement Phase you gain the clarity to integrate them within the total picture. Exercise selection evolves into a gem-cutter's sophistication in the program design of your health and strength (and that of your clients).

You begin to refurbish your *Mental Blueprint* and as a result paint an accurate picture of you interwoven in your environment. It is no longer the heavy power tools, but now careful maintenance, vigilant care, and (most importantly) relaxed enjoyment of the work you have done that are important. It is not vanity or decoration, but more a Feng Shui approach to your Self-Image.

Skill Development Stages

The Recover-Coordination-Refinement process relates precisely to motor science. Psychologist Paul Fitts commented on 3 stages to learning a new skill (Thomas David Kehoe, 1997):

Cognitive: in which you learn the performance goals of the skill. You must consciously regulate and control each skill nuance.

Associative: in which you perform the skill. Your skill timing and rhythm refine unconsciously, increasing fluidity.

Autonomous: in which your skill becomes automatic and unconscious.

In the cognitive phase you concentrate on the integration of three physical virtues: breathing, movement, and structure. Pay attention to detail. In the associative stage you no longer need to concentrate on the external performance goals of the skill in order to regulate the movement. Attention transforms into effort. Effort regards the internal sensation of your skill performance goals. Feel the outcome of each performance goal inside of you. In the associative stage you begin a "program" of *Biomechanical Exercise* because only through a program can you actually begin to refine the skill to its final stage.

In the autonomous stage, you refine the skill to the level of unconscious performance. Begin to alter effort protocol to challenge your persistence. You reap the greatest benefits in this stage because you can achieve the greatest intensity and depth of concentration here. You push the envelope and increase the threshold of your capabilities. You open up and reveal your **Body-Flow**!

STEPS FOR DEEPENING YOUR DAILY PRACTICE OF *BODY-FLOW*

First and foremost, establish a safe, clean and quiet practice environment. Sweep your practice area before you begin and ensure no obstacles lay in the path of your movements.

Take the time to sit down and clear your head before your session. Tell your self that it can resume thoughts about the so-called "important things" when you're through with your practice.

Do some deep, full Performance Breathing exhalations for two minutes before beginning.

Pull out your Practice Dairy and review the three *Biomechanical Exercise*s you have chosen to weave into a Kinetic Chain.

Practice the components of the 1st *Biomechanical Exercise* as a 5-minute warm-up. Make certain that each component properly integrates your breathing, movement and structure.

Yield to the excess tensions you feel. Do not force your self through any bracing, wincing or flinching. Allow the tension to melt away by going even more slowly. Use only that tension necessary to maintain structure, facilitate breathing and cause the intended motion.

Compose the components into a *Biomechanical Exercise* Work ultra-slow ensuring that the transition between each component meshes seamlessly.

As you start to move faster in your *Biomechanical Exercise* view tension as a "pressure cooker." Always reduce never increase the pressure. Speed should occur due to unconscious efficiency.

Keep exploring the *Biomechanical Exercise* until you can perform it with no conscious involvement, or until 30 minutes have lapsed. If less than 30 min. pass then…

Begin with the components of the 2nd *Biomechanical Exercise* and repeat steps 5 – 9.

Begin with the components of the 3rd *Biomechanical Exercise* and repeat steps 5 – 9.

Take the ending component of the 1st *Biomechanical Exercise* and graft it to the beginning component of the 2nd. Work ultra-slow ensuring that the transition between each component meshes seamlessly.

Practice the 1st and 2nd *Biomechanical Exercise*s as one movement to create your first Kinetic Chain. Keep exploring the Kinetic Chain until you can perform it with no conscious involvement.

Take the ending component of the 2nd *Biomechanical Exercise* and graft it to the beginning component of the 3rd. Work ultra-slow ensuring that the transition between each component meshes seamlessly.

Practice the 2nd and 3rd *Biomechanical Exercise*s as one movement and explore it until you can perform it with no conscious involvement.

Practice all three *Biomechanical Exercise*s as one movement and explore the complete Kinetic Chain until you can perform it with no conscious involvement.

Restrict your sessions to no more than 40 minutes per day.

KEY POINTS AND PERFORMANCE GOALS

Never begin exercise without specific permission for this type of exercise from your physician.

Never practice a movement that will adversely affect a pre-existing injury or condition.

Certain patterns of *Fear-Reactivity* can produce "performance anxiety" about getting the movements "absolutely correct." Do not fixate on the "ideal concepts" of the movements. Rather, explore the flow of the movements. You cannot think your way to more efficient movement, structure and breathing.

Don't fixate on your mistakes. Let them go and move along. You do not need to stop and record in your Diary mistakes.

Practice Diaries should be "reflections" not reports. Immediately after the session, do a 5-minute stream of consciousness. Don't prejudice, just let the words flow out.

Change your Kinetic Chains or *Biomechanical Exercises* as you feel like it. Variety can add spice! Have Fun!

CONCLUSION

By writing this book, I experienced a great catharsis, a lifetime release. I had worried that I would never be able to present in a distilled version, the essence of all that I have learned in my years traveling and fighting across the world, studying and researching with the brightest minds in many disciplines, learning and exploring in my own "Mountain laboratories."

I honestly doubted that I would be able to write so succinctly and maintain the purity and comprehensiveness of the message. However, my pleasure in this final product exceeds any that I had experienced in all my other works. It may become my *Magnus opus*, my primary contribution to the world.

In a way, I may have surprised your expectations. You may have thought that you purchased a book on fitness and conditioning, or on movement performance – coordination, agility, balance. What you received was so much more, so much deeper and impacting than that facsimile - the socially programmed definition of personal image.

You received a book on *Form*. **Body-Flow** regards no shape, but the essence of what it is to be you. By revealing the underlying "you" ensconced under that veneer of socially imposed definition, you discover that you always and already are masterful.

For me, this book revealed some interesting discoveries about my current condition as a "celebrity." My name now holds weight. Read that again. My name is now heavy… attached. People associate me with certain ideas, principles and works. They identify me with symbols, logos and slogans.

But I am not those things. I am not those attachments. *I am not those addictions.* I am greater than the sum of my experiences. What I have experienced provided me with the opportunity ONLY to distill who I am, to BE myself in the midst of greater and greater crisis and challenge.

This may very well be my final work I publish. I'm not sure at this time. A very long time ago, one of the wisest men I had ever had the honor of knowing, Doctor Jonathon Ellsworth Winter, said to me, *"Philosophy is essentially a degenerative pursuit. The more you bring order to world, the more you impose artificiality on that which is authentic and pure."*

I know that **Body-Flow** was my most challenging task to date. My goal was to craft this content and compose the words in such a way that it brought the opportunity for freedom, not increased entrapment to you. It is not an attempt to impose upon you an order of things, but rather it gives you the doorway to your authenticity and purity.

The material herein does not intend to become dogma. I expect a few of you out there who read this and resonate with its message will sally forth into new jungles. I expect that some of you in the future will take this material and go farther than I did.

This is why I used the quote from Descartes' Error, "I am skeptical of science's presumption of objectivity and definitiveness. I have a difficult time seeing scientific result as anything but provisional approximations, to be enjoyed for a while and discarded as soon as better accounts become available." (Damasio)

Currently, I know that there is no other presentation or system that provides such an opportunity for depth to so many people like *Body-Flow*. There's simply nothing comparable in any discipline, nor in any three combined. But I hope that changes because of my book!

Read *Body-Flow* and allow it to transform your life; allow it to be the boat to cross the river rapids of your *Fear-Reactivity*; allow it to return you to the shores of your inherent talent, genius and abundance, and to the forests of your unlimited health, strength and performance.

But don't view the exercises contained in this book as the penultimate. I selected these from the thousands I created in my system. But more than that, *Body-Flow* is an underpinning purpose to all physical movement in general. It's not a program, it's a schema. It's a way of looking and interfacing with the world, and rejoining the natural flow of everything… it's a way of removing the final wall – the distinction between you and the world.

Go deeply.

Scott Sonnon

APPENDIX I:
BASIC STRUCTURES OF BIOMECHANICAL EXERCISE

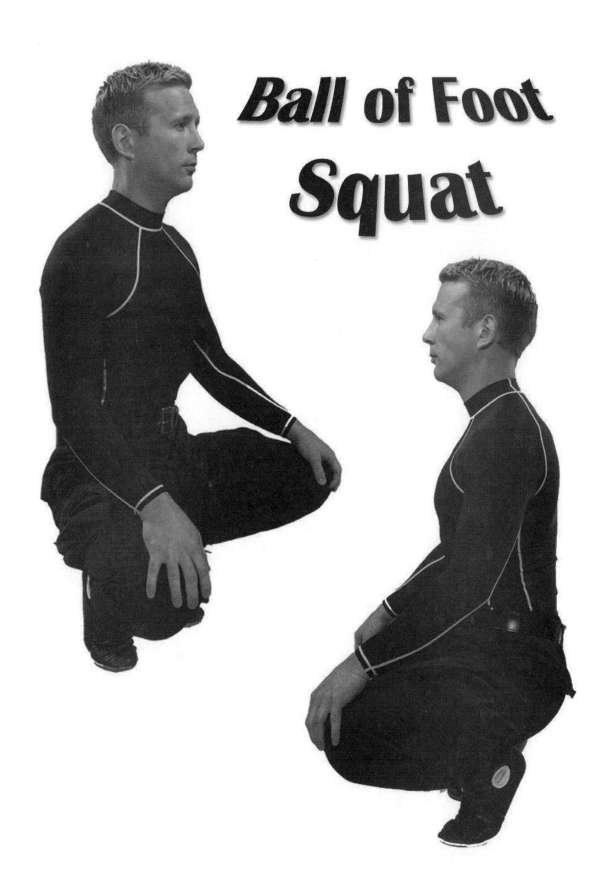

Ball of Foot Squat

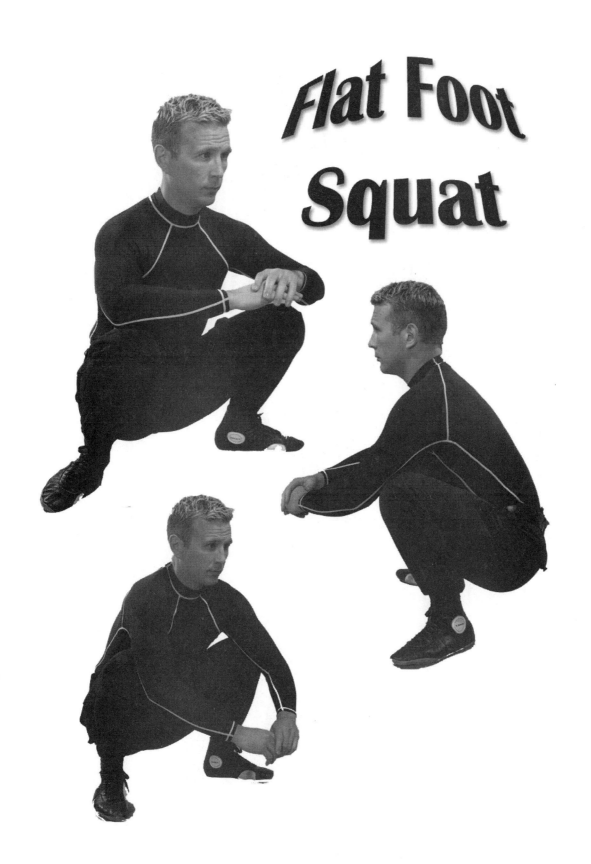

Flat Foot Squat

Cossack Squat

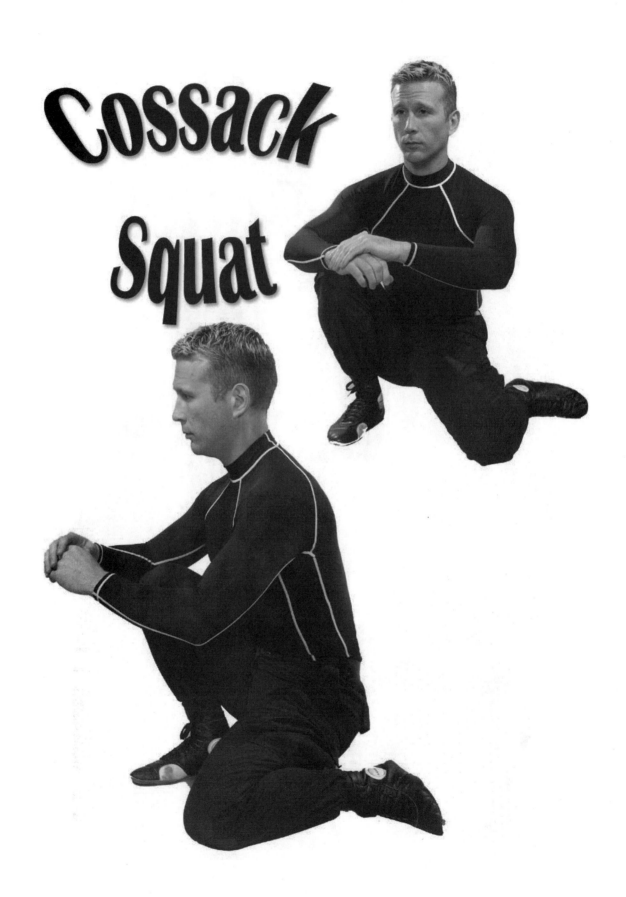

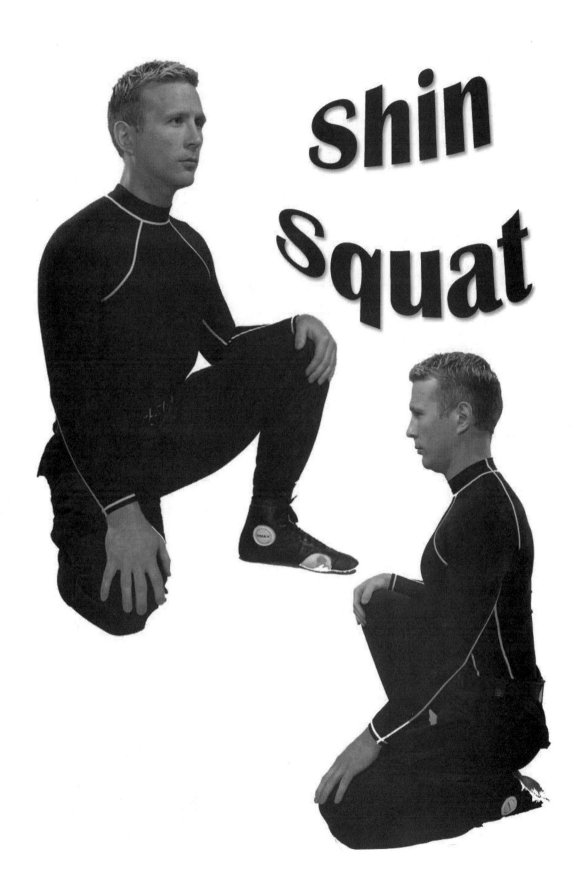

Shin Squat

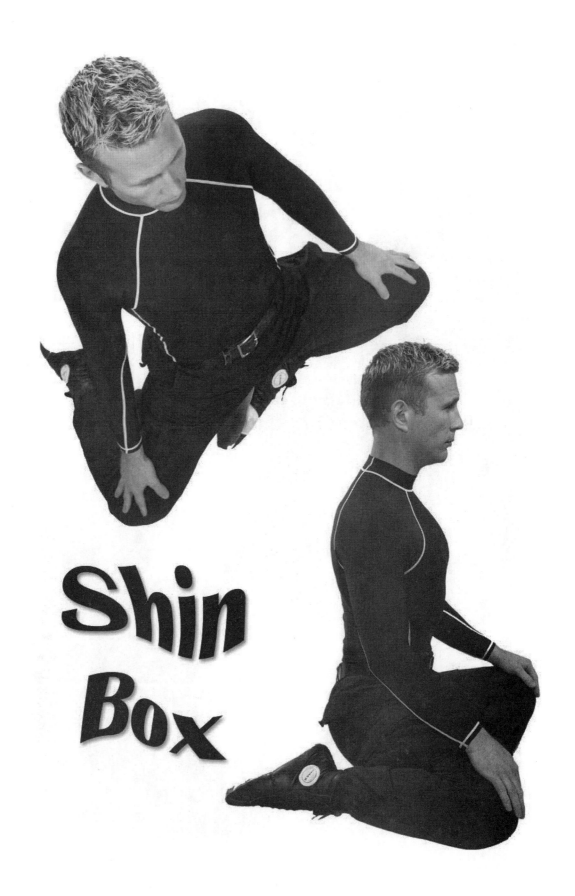

Shin
Box

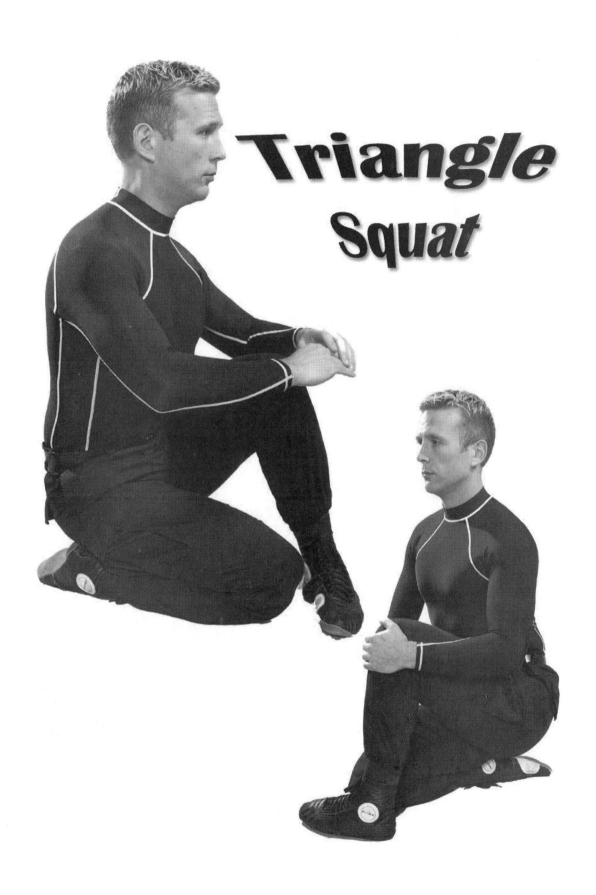

Triangle Squat

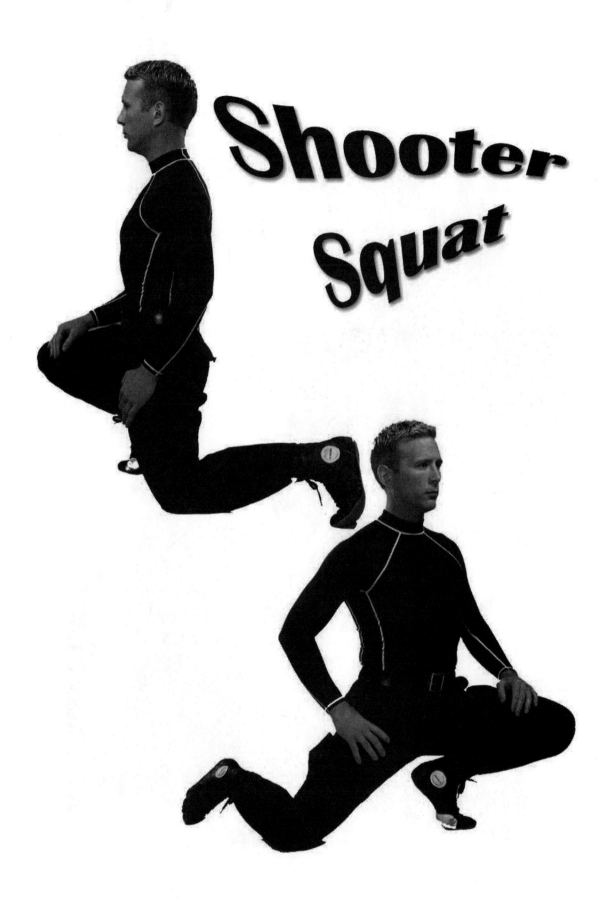

Shooter Squat

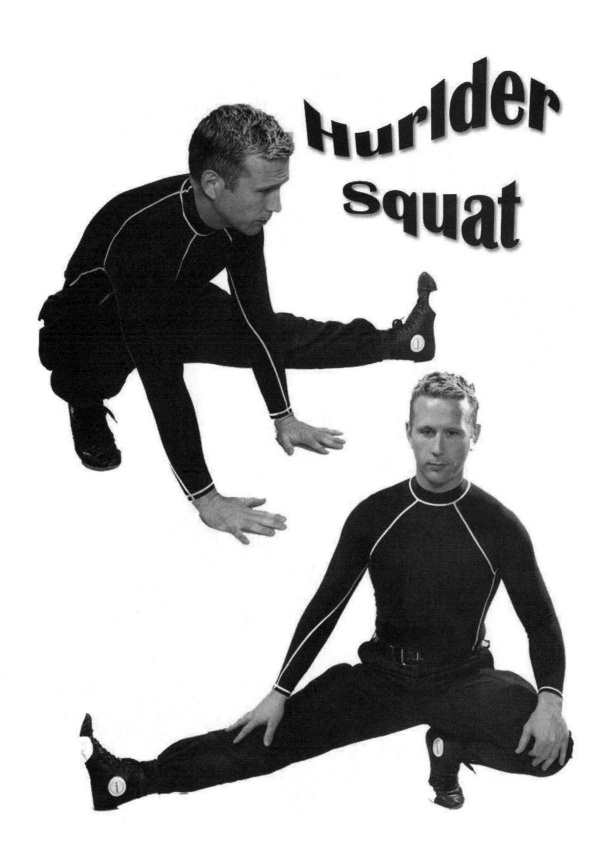

Hurlder Squat

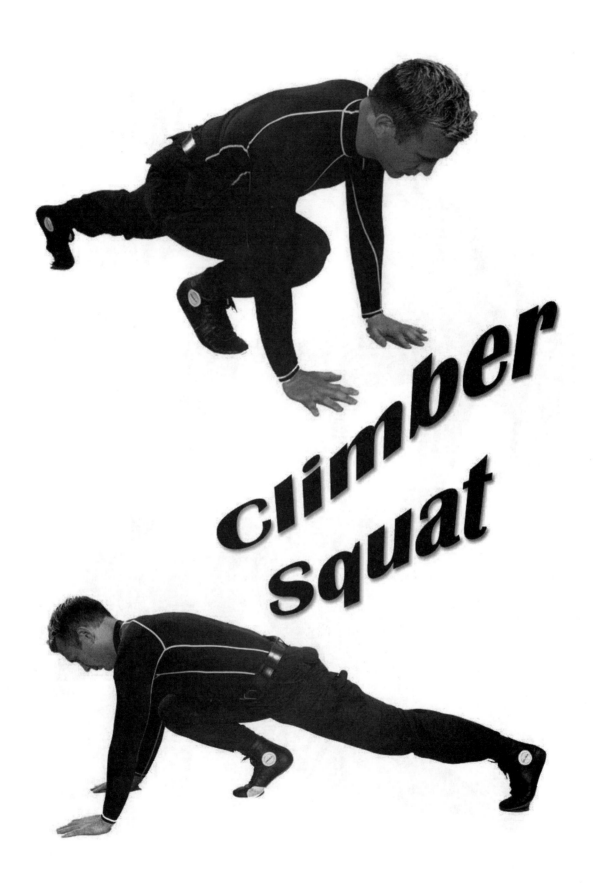

climber
squat

Quad Squat

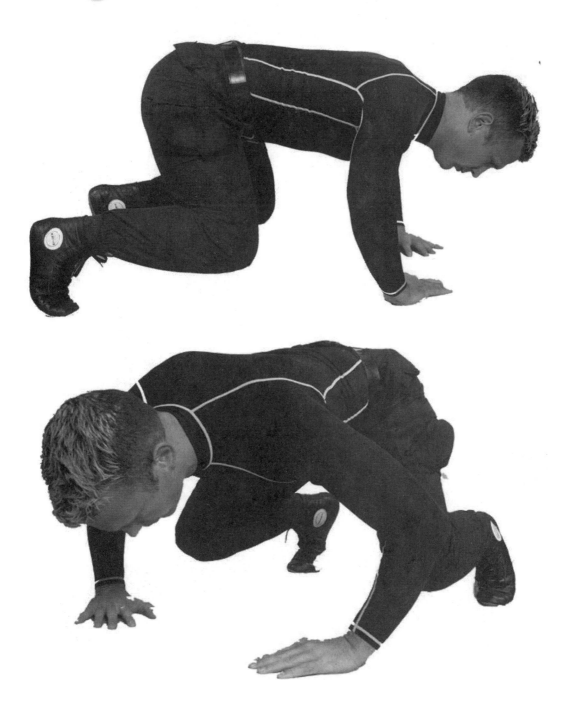

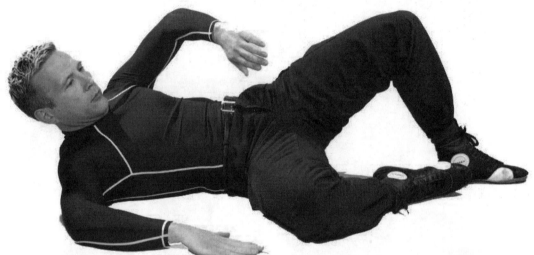

Position of Assurance

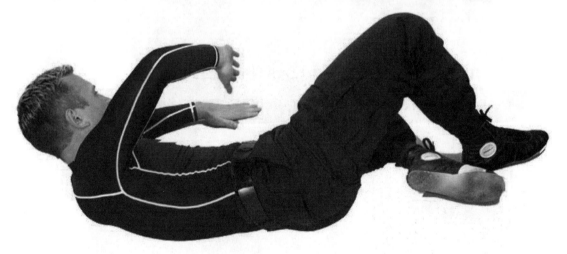

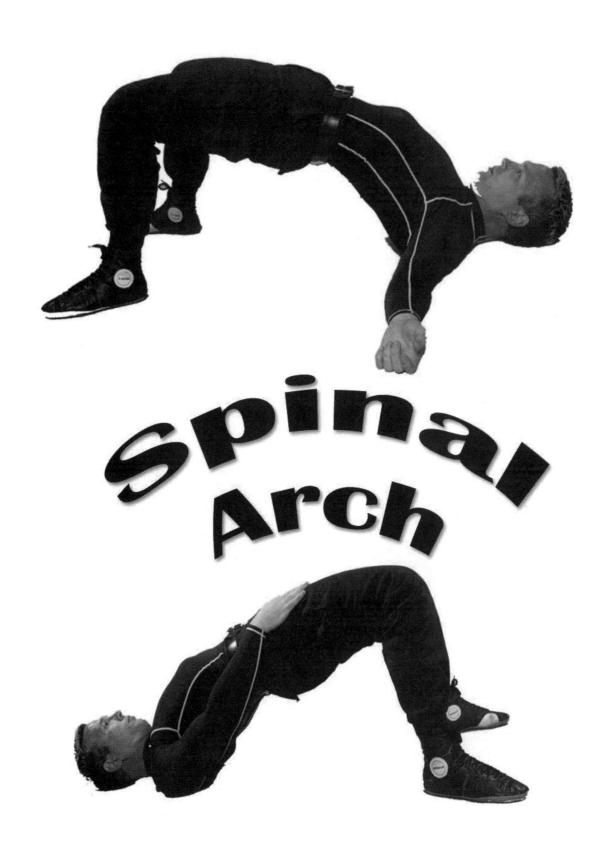

Spinal Arch

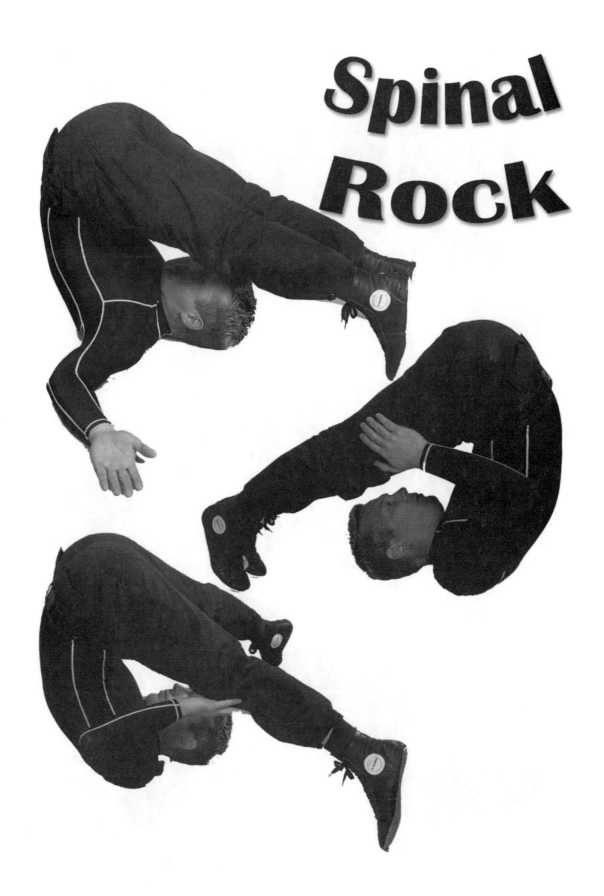

Spinal Rock

APPENDIX II:
SELECTION OF BIOMECHANICAL EXERCISE FOR BODY-FLOW

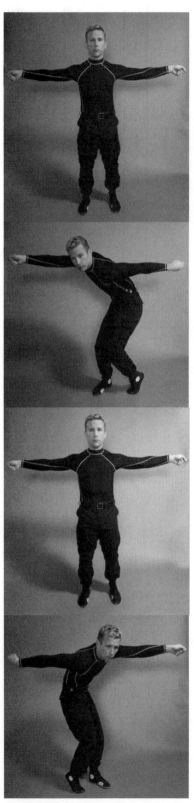

Arm Screw

Begin with arms straight outward.

Exhale and rotate your entire arm forward.

Allow your hips to move outwards slightly.

Allow the same knee of the rotating shoulder to dip inward.

Keep arms directly parallel to the floor at all times, as if your arms were tethered in opposite directions.

Roll your shoulder backward and assume an upright posture again.

Switch and do the same with the opposite shoulder.

When done correctly your motion breathes you.

With refinement you shall discover the roots of one of my breathing techniques called *Alternating Breath*: which involves compressing one lung and breathing with the opposite, then switching.

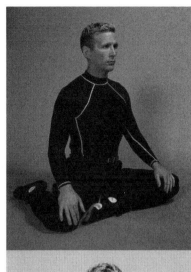

Shinbox Switch

Begin in Shinbox position.

Exhale and curve your spine backward, as you allow your knees to simultaneously lift upwards.

Keep your feet on the ground at all times; don't adjust your footing.

Continue through the Seated Position without pause.

Inhale as your chest expands when you drop your knees downward into the opposite Shinbox.

Feel yourself pulled from the crown of your head as if being hung like a string of pearls.

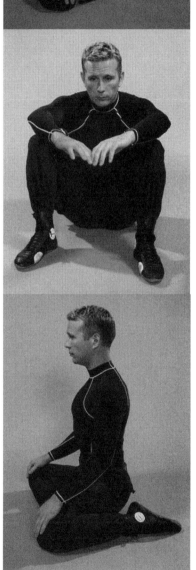

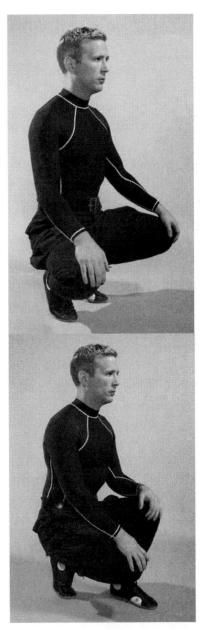

Squat Creep

Begin in Ball of Foot Squat position.

Allow your weight to transfer to one foot.

With your free leg step forward only far enough to place your foot flat on the ground.

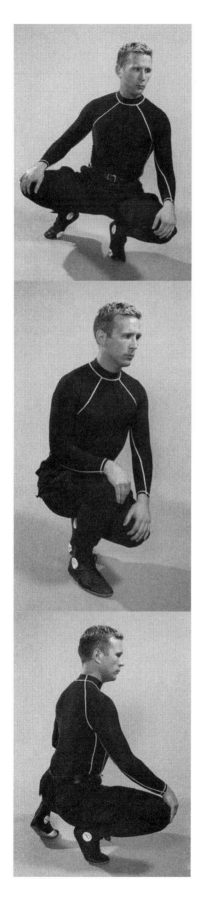

As you shift your weight onto the advanced leg, draw your opposite knee backwards (without moving its planted foot – only pivot.)

Use the pivot of the back knee movement to CREATE the forward weight transfer.

With your weight balanced on the forward leg, step linearly (not swinging circularly) forward until your foot becomes flat on the ground. Repeat!

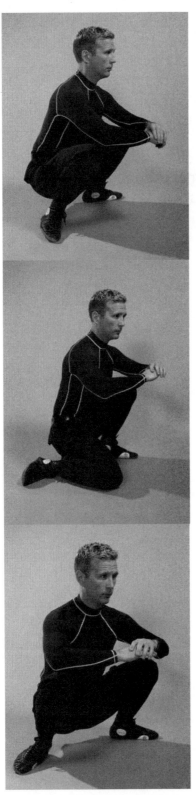

Knee Switch

Begin in Flat Foot Squat position.

Allow the inside of one knee to drop so that your shin firmly confirms the entire surface of the ground.

Don't strain your knee. Allow your hip to push your dropping knee a bit forward en route to the ground.

Always keep your heel (and entire foot) in contact with the ground as you drop your knee. You should relax into this position without strain.

You arrive in the Cossack Squat!

To lift your knee, merely shift your hips and weight transfer off of the flat foot to un-weight the dropped knee. It should be light and effortless to return back to the Ball of Foot Squat.

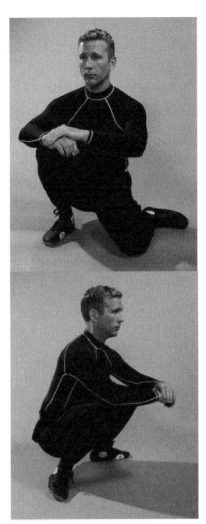

Switch and Repeat! Effortlessly flow from one side alternating with the next!

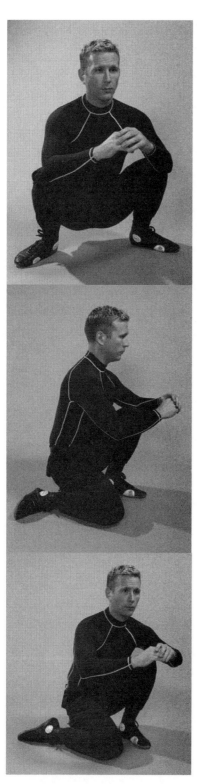

Shin Roll

Begin in Flat Foot Squat.

Drop your knee as in the Knee Switch to arrive in a Cossack Squat.

Shift your weight parallel to the ground by rolling your bottom over your shin.

Keep your instep (top of foot) in contact with the ground at all times.

Curl your toes under as if pointing them, and you pass through the Shin Squat.

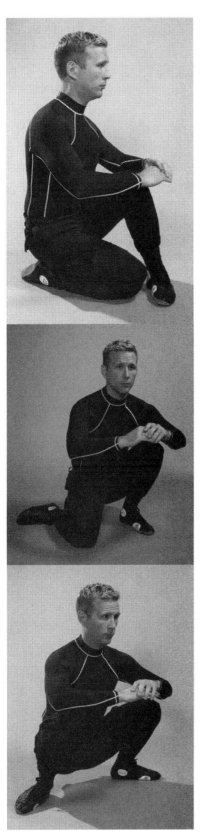

Roll your weight completely around, letting the knee of the planted shin pivot to your opposite foot – arriving at a Triangle Squat.

To reverse the motion, swing your hips around the direction they came, un-weighting your shin and transferring your weight to your opposite foot.

Once your weight completely frees from the planted shin, un-point your toes, flexing them into an L-shaped position of the Cossack Squat.

As in the Knee Switch, simply rotate the pelvis and weight transfer off of your planted foot to lift the planted shin effortlessly.

You arrive back in the Flat Foot Squat.

Now Switch to the other leg and repeat back and forth, alternating in one fluid motion.

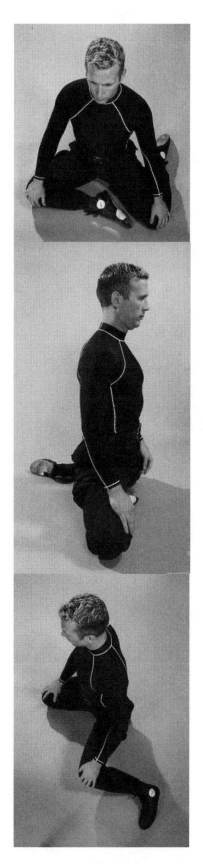

Standing Shinroll
Begin in the Shinbox.

Expand your hips and roll onto your front shin.

Keep your toes pointed and the top of your foot flush with the ground.

With your weight transferred to your front shin, you can swing around your rear leg in a tight circle.

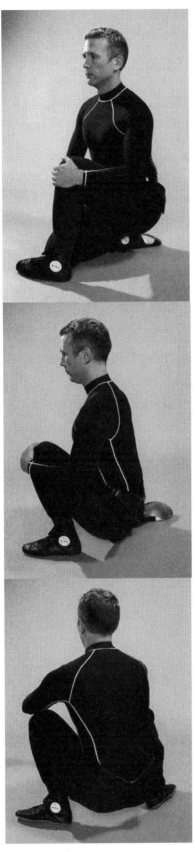

Placing the inside of your swinging foot perpendicular to your planted shin, you arrive at the Triangle Squat.

Keeping the motion continuing, allow your weight to transfer to your newly planted flat foot.

Roll the heel of your planted shin to the ground and curl your toes towards.

You pass through the Shin Squat and translate immediately towards the Cossack Squat.

Lift your knee by rotating your pelvis a la Knee Switch, and you arrive in the Flat Foot Squat!

You can continue from here by gently falling back into the same Shinbox and repeating, or you may drop into the opposite Shinbox and proceed in the obverse direction.

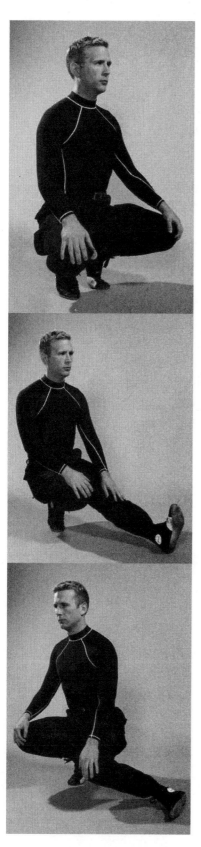

Long Leg Creep

Begin in the Ball of Foot Squat.

Shift your weight to one Ball of Foot, to free the opposite leg.

Maintaining your balance extend your leg so that the heel touches the ground and your knee is nearly locked.

You arrive in a forward Hurdler Squat.

Rotate your knee inward and towards the ground as if moving towards a Cossack Squat or Shinroll.

As you do, shift your weight to the back leg.

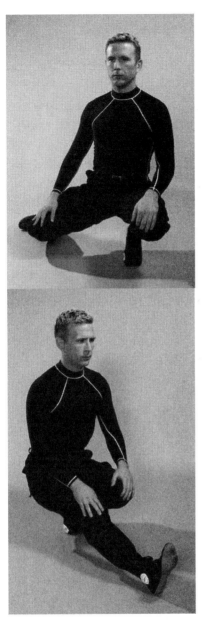

Perform a Knee Switch and transfer your weight to your front leg arriving in a Shooter Squat.

Shift all of your weight to your front leg and step through with your back leg to continue the Long Leg Creep.

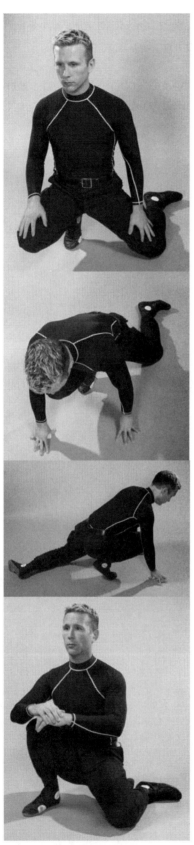

Shin Swing

From a Shooter Squat, lean (don't bend) forward and place your hands on the ground.

Using your hands, spin on your Ball of Foot plant backwards.

Keep your downed shin parallel to the ground, and your heel downward (as if in Cossack Squat).

Once you rotate 180 degrees (or actually whatever you wish), gently push back off of your hands to transfer your weight to your back leg.

You arrive in the Cossack Squat.

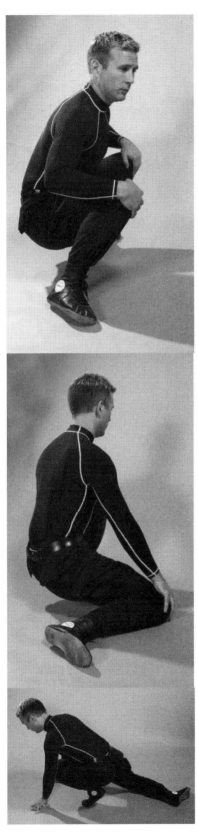

Lift your knee as in the Knee Switch.

Drop your opposite knee and arrive in the opposite Cossack Squat.

Transfer your weight forward onto your front Ball of Foot to arrive in the Shooter Squat.

Place your hands on the ground and pivot backwards on the Ball of Foot of your front leg.

Repeat and continue alternating legs!

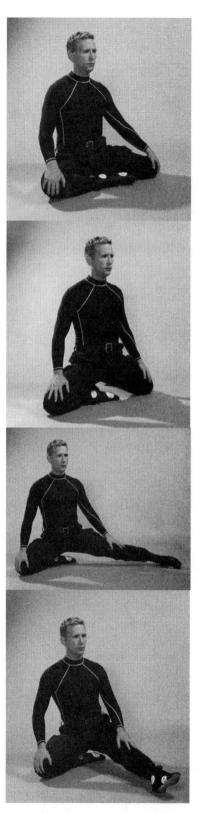

Double Shin Roll

Begin in the Shinbox.

Elevate your hip to free the back leg, a la Standing Shinroll.

Keep your swinging leg as long to your side as possible.

Swing your leg in a large arc until it is directly in front of you.

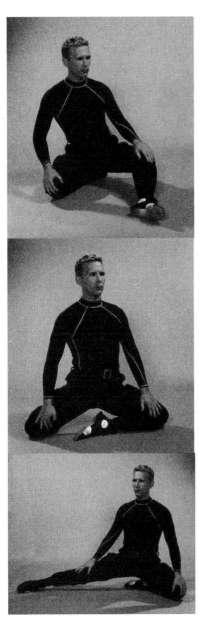

Bend your forward knee and begin weight transferring off of your back shin.

Roll your forward shin to arrive in a Elevated Shinbox.

Repeat on the opposite leg!

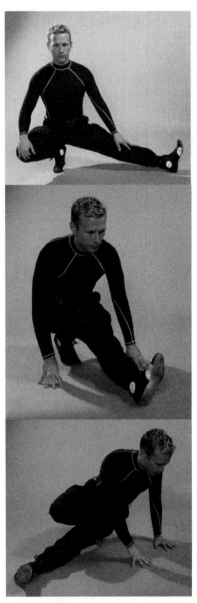

Leg Swoop

Begin in the Hurdler Squat and swing your lengthened leg around in front of you.

Continue the swing towards your planted Ball of Foot and place both of your hands to the outside of the swinging leg.

Weight transfer onto your hands and free your back leg.

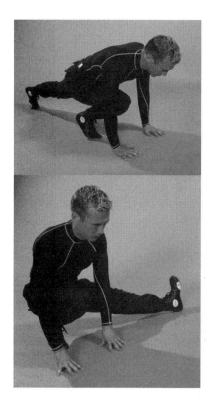

Continue the Swing by hopping over your swinging leg with your back leg.

You arrive in the Climber Squat.

Continue the motion uninterrupted to return the beginning step.

Continue the motion in one large circle to complete the exercise.

Practice placing your hands as lightly on the ground as possible and swing your leg as fluidly as possible.

Elevated Scorpion

Begin in Lateral Hurdler Squat.

Rotate your hands in front of you towards the knee of your planted foot.

You arrive in a Climber Squat.

Shift your weight off of your planted foot and distribute the weight between your hands and your extended leg.

Lift your planted leg in a diagonal arc up towards the opposite shoulder.

Lift your knee as high towards your head as possible.

Keep your extended leg in one point at all times.

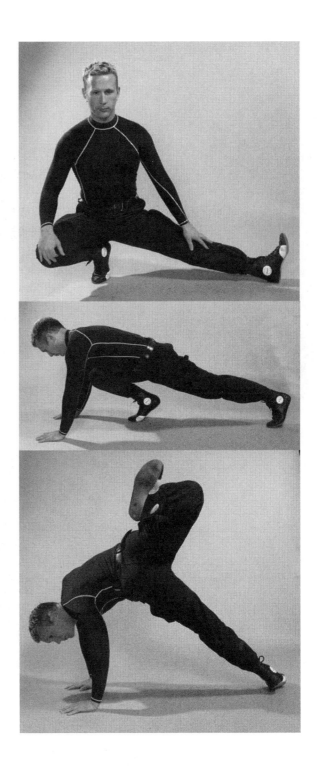

Allow your elevated leg to carry you over releasing the arm on the same side of the elevated leg.

Continue the momentum of the movement and you arrive in a Hurdler Squat.

Initially brace yourself by placing your hands on the ground to stop the motion. Work to land in Hurdler Squat with no hands.

Use your extended leg as the pivot point to continue the exercise in a complete circle of revolving Elevated Scorpions.

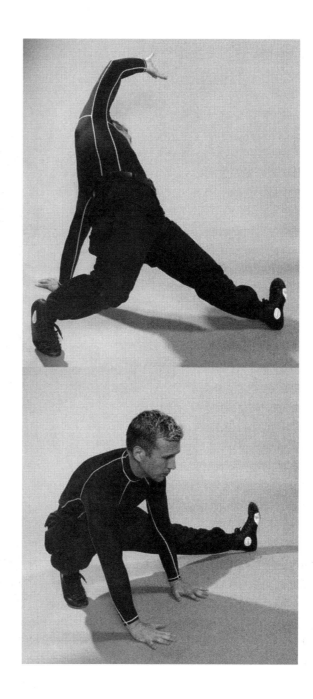

Long Leg Roll

Begin with your knees at chest and shins flat on the ground.

Extend one leg with pointed toes.

The same shoulder should rotate forward towards the ground.

Exhale as the movement compresses your lungs.

Slide your hips off of the remaining leg underneath.

Roll your top shoulder upwards and over so that you arrive on your back.

Draw your extended leg upwards to match the leg which remained knee to chest.

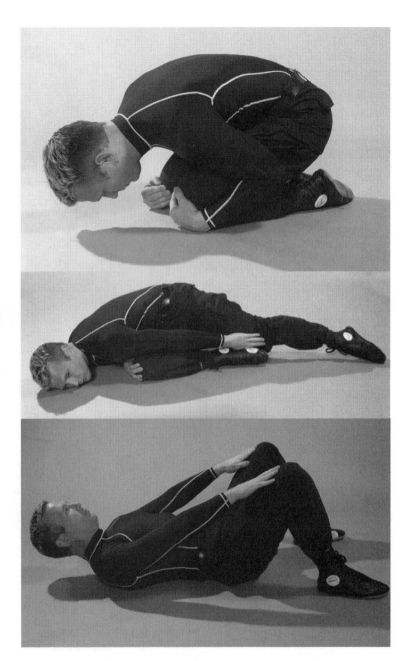

Continuing in the same direction, draw the opposite knee to your chest as you extend the opposite leg.

Remember to roll the shoulder (on the same side as the extended leg) towards the ground and exhale.

Use the momentum gained from extending your leg to roll yourself on top of the shin which remained at your chest.

Continuing the motion draw the extended leg underneath to arrive at the beginning.

Repeat and continue with fluidity.

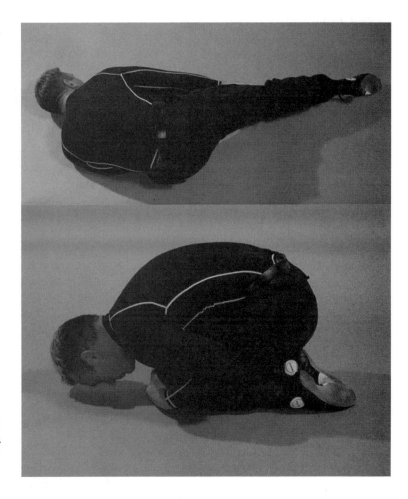

Leg Thread

Begin in Position of Assurance.

Slide your planted elbow upwards beyond your head.

Simultaneously slide your planted shin with toes pointed behind your planted foot. This exposes your side to the ground.

As you continue, place your top hand down on the ground and continue to slide your elbow upward as you turn downward.

Extend long with your threading leg to expose the front of your hips to the ground.

Continue the motion by bringing your opposite knee underneath the leg which you just extended.

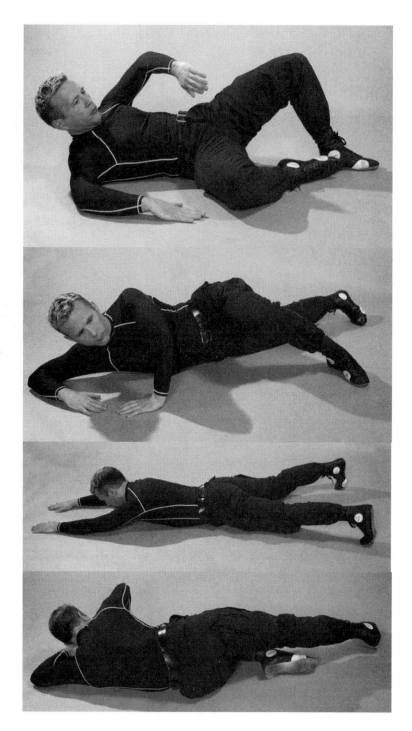

Slide your bottom arm
down towards your
ribs, and you return to
the Position of
Assurance.

Roll your top shoulder
back and down to the
ground, fluidly
switching your arm
position, and
exchanging your top
knee down and your
bottom knee up.

Repeat and Continue!

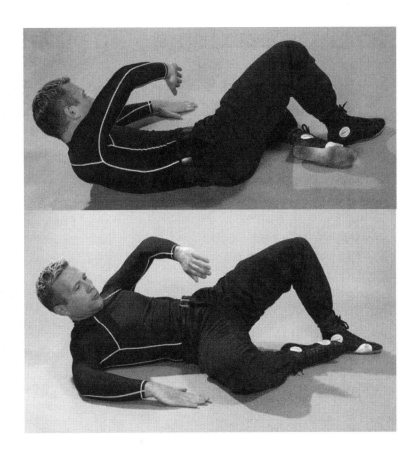

Double Leg Swoop

Begin in the Position of Assurance.

Move your top leg across your bottom leg as far as you can reach.

Exhale as this compresses your diaphragm.

Begin to swing your top leg in a larch arch across your body.

Exhale deeper into the swing.

Once you begin the swing, your hips (Lunar Plexus) should free, and your weight should transfer to your Solar Plexus.

Allow your mobile hips to swing your bottom leg in tandem chasing but never advancing upon your top leg.

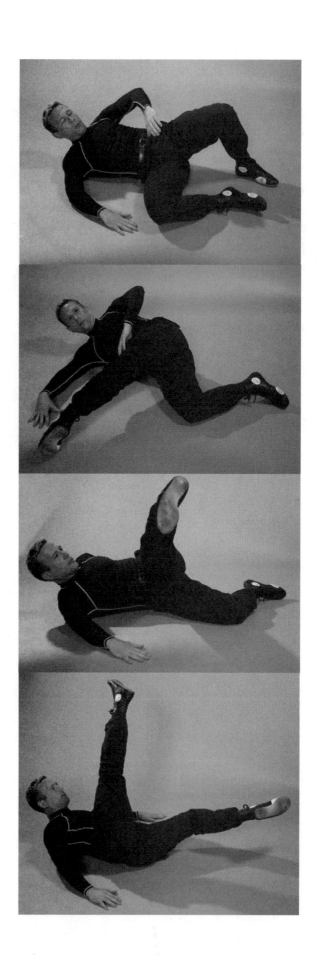

Move your top leg over as far as possible.

Allow your bottom leg to thread under the new top leg.

Extend your arms above your torso to expose your front to the ground.

Lift the opposite leg to begin a second revolution of the Double Leg Swoop, or to end in Position of Assurance.

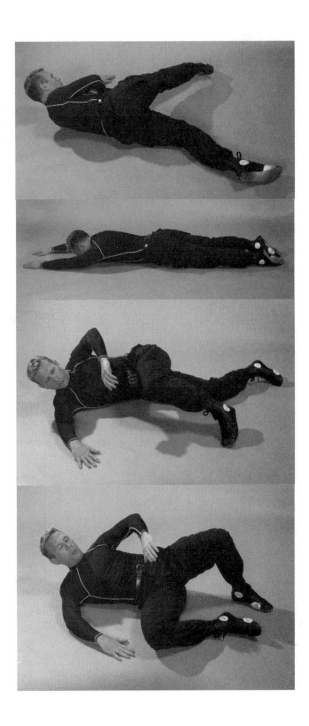

Arching Leg Thread

Begin in Spinal Arch with your elbows pinched to your ribs and your hands by your chin.

Thread your leg underneath while maintaining the arch.

Reach deep with the threading leg to expose your front to the ground.

Transfer your weight to your forearms, and the balls of your feet.

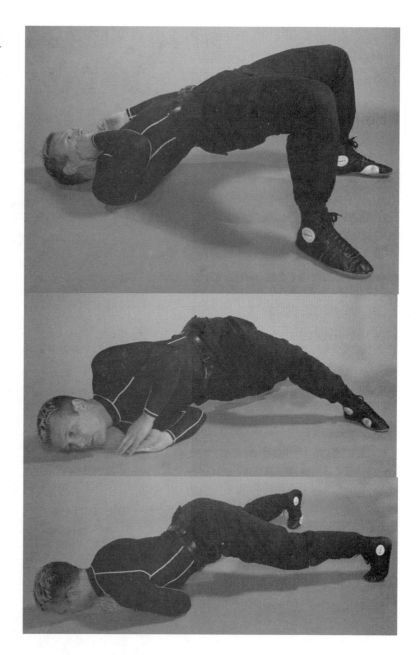

Shift your weight to one forearm, freeing the top shoulder to roll upward and around towards the ground.

Thread the opposite leg under, while maintaining the Spinal Arch.

You arrive at the Spinal Arch again!

Repeat and Continue in a circle!

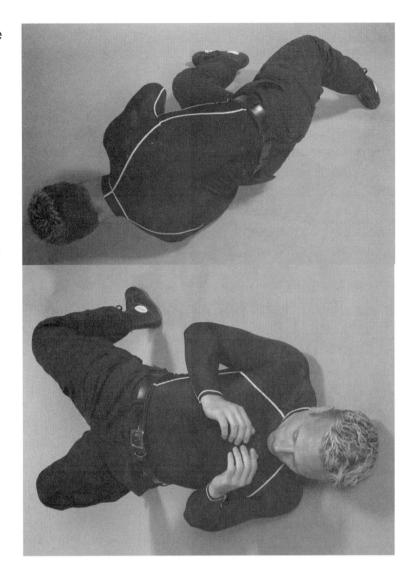

Spinal Rock

Begin in a Seated Ready Position.

Begin arching your spine backward and tucking your pelvis upward so that your spine becomes rounded.

Rolling backwards with your chin tucked exhale as you fully compress your lungs.

Rock back and project your Solar Plexus upwards.

Inhale as you lengthen your spine as if lifting the crown hanging by a string.

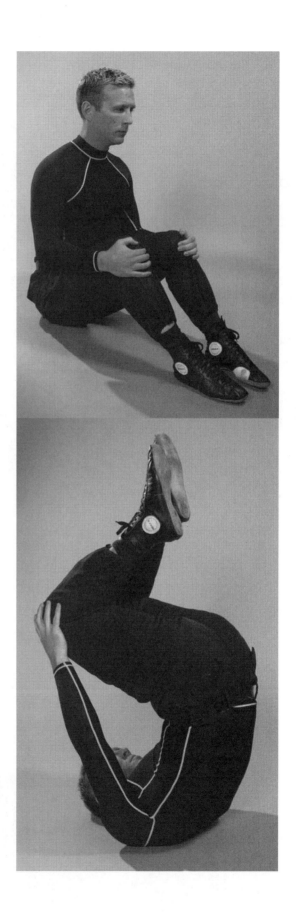

Spinal Rock: Extended Pike

Begin in a Seated Ready Position with legs extended and together.

Roll backward bringing knees close.

When on your shoulder blades exhale and extend your legs upward.

Bring your knees back to your chest and return to Seated Ready.

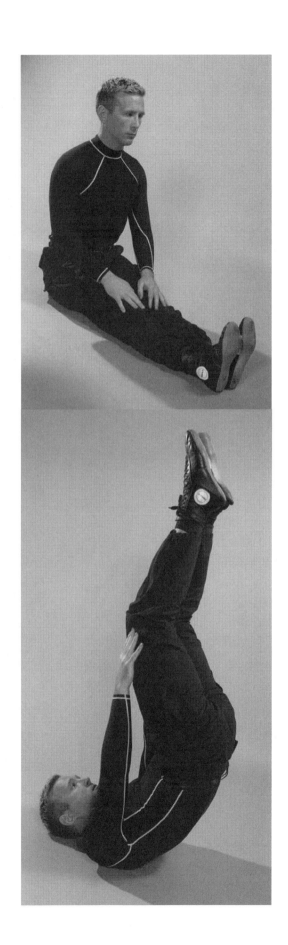

Spinal Rock: Straddle Split

Begin in a Seated Ready Position with legs extended outward.

Keep your spine lifted upwards from your crown.

Exhale and roll backward bringing knees to the sides of your head.

When on your shoulder blades exhale and lock your knees gently.

Relax your knees back to your chest and return to Straddle Split as you inhale and extend your spine.

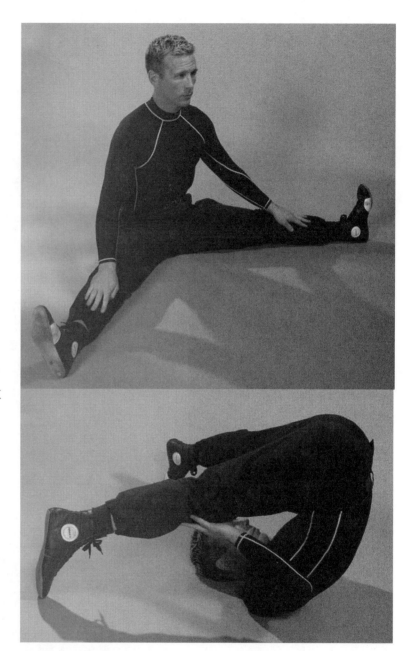

Spinal Rock: Hurdler Split

Begin in a Seated Ready Position with one leg extended forward and the other tucked in a la Shinbox.

Keep your spine lifted upwards from your crown.

Exhale and roll backward bringing your extended leg back over your head to touch the ground while your tuck.

When on your shoulder blades exhale and lock your extended knee gently.

Relax your knee back to your chest.

Keep your originally tucked leg extended and tuck your originally extended leg to land in the opposite Hurdler Split.

Repeat and continue alternating!

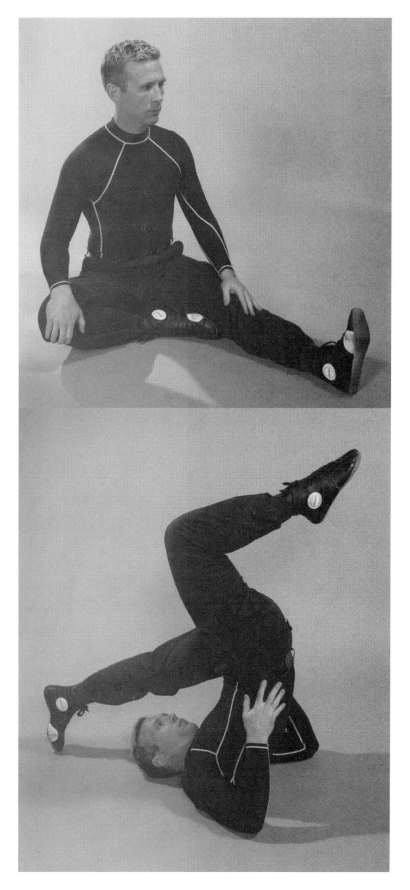

Spinal Rock: Shinbox

Begin in Shinbox.

Exhale and roll backward bringing your Shinbox above your head.

When on your shoulder blades exhale and TWIST your Shinbox into the opposite Shinbox over head.

Relax the new structure to your chest and land in the ORIGINAL Shinbox structure.

Repeat and continue!

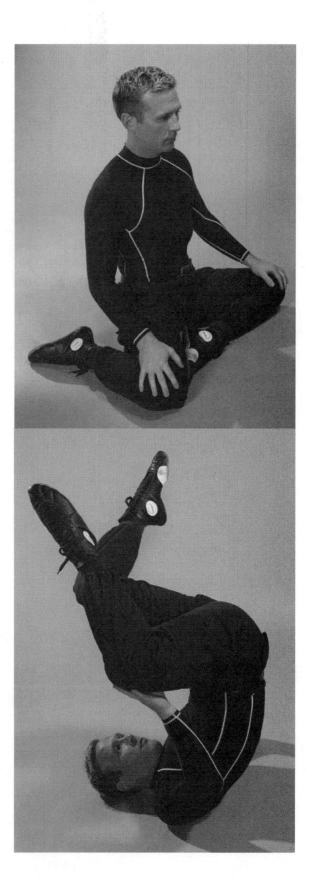

Spinal Rock: Butterfly

Begin in a Seated Ready Position with feet together and knees pressed downward.

Keep your spine lifted upwards from your crown.

Exhale and roll backward bringing knees to the sides of your head while keeping the soles of your feet together.

When on your shoulder blades extend your hips.

Relax your hips downward and return to Butterfly as you inhale and extend your spine.

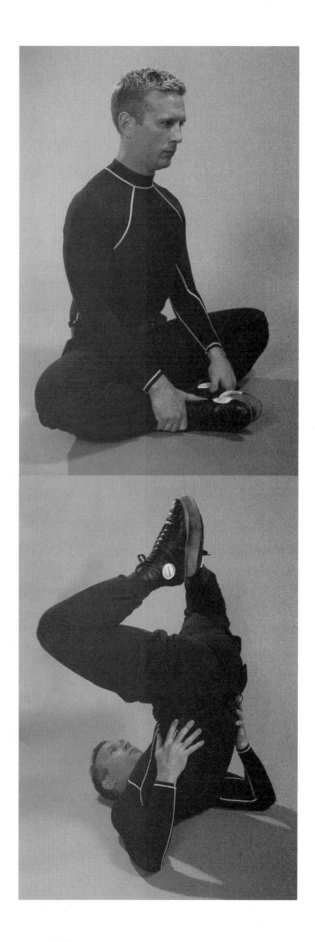

Swing Split

Begin in Ball of Foot Squat.

Lean to the side and place your near hand directly downward.

Simultaneously extend your legs: bottom leg forward and top leg backward.

Extend your top arm and open your chest as you inhale.

Relax and exhale as you bend your knees back underneath you.

Press off of your planted hand to weight transfer back into a Ball of Foot Squat.

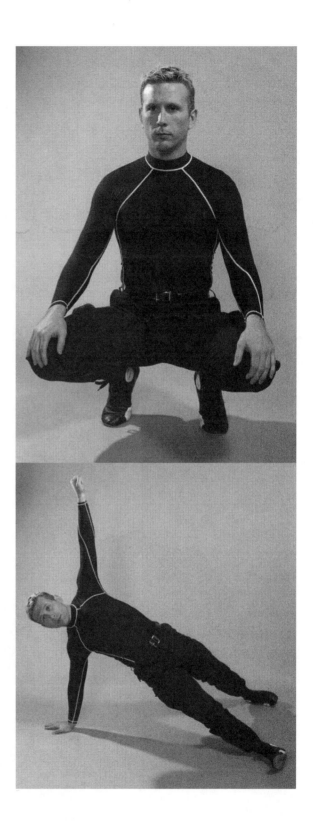

OR you can modify the Ball of Foot Squat by adding forward hand placement.

Immediately continue the motion by leaning to the opposite side.

Place the near hand on the ground and repeat on the opposite side.

Alternate and Continue!

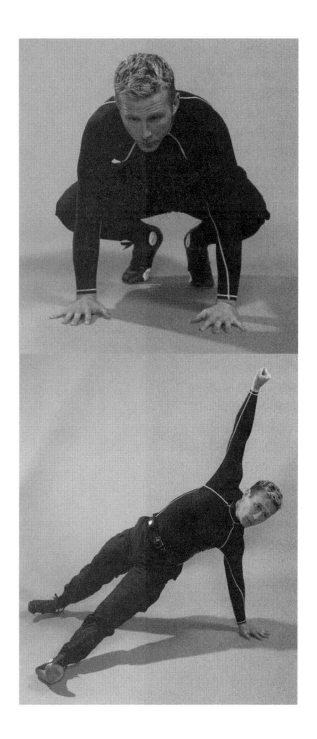

Quad Switch

Begin in Quad Squat.

Lift opposite arm and leg while keep proper structure and your spine parallel to the ground.

Thread your lifted knee underneath the diagonal line as you allow your free shoulder to swing backward.

Continue backward and place your hand on the ground where your lifted foot once planted, and your foot where your lifted hand once planted.

You land in a Reverse Quad Squat.

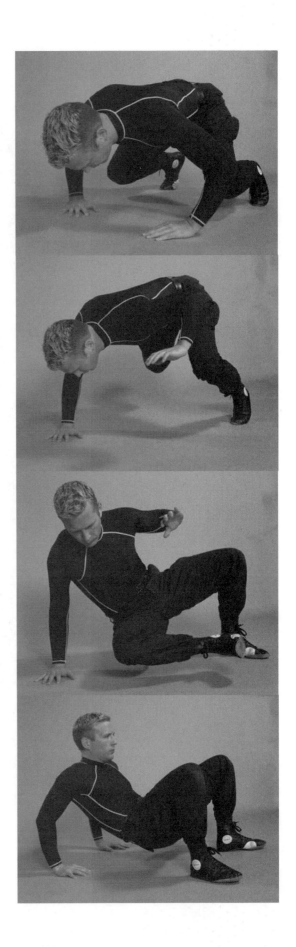

Lift the opposite arm and leg combo.

Thread the lifting foot underneath as you reach over with the free hand.

Return to the original Quad Squat.

Repeat fluidly and continue with as little pause between steps as possible!

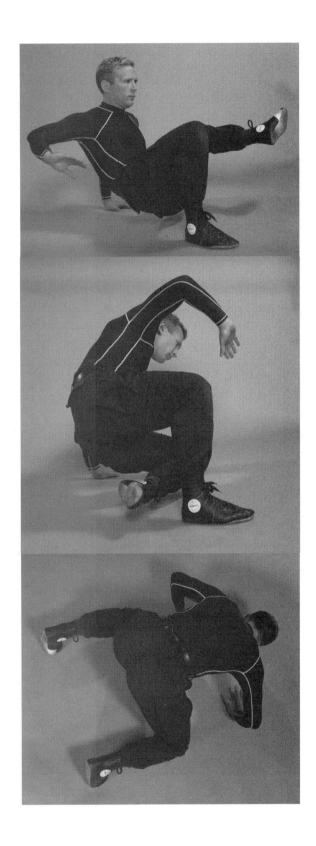

Long Arm Roll

Begin in a Cossack Squat with an Arm Screw. The shoulder rolling downwards should be over the knee of the planted shin. Exhale.

Exhale further as you roll UNDER not over your shoulder. Keep screwing the shoulder underneath.

Your heel of the planted shin should lift as you begin to screw yourself under (not over!)

Use the opposite hand to plant. Look closely at the hand structure.

Tuck your chin and move your head underneath your free armpit. Exhale.

Only your back (NOT YOUR NECK OR SHOULDER!) should touch the ground.

Do not LEAP! Roll UNDER!

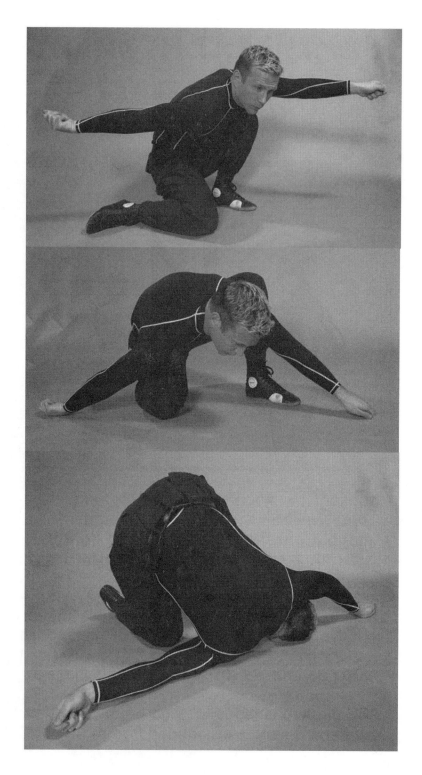

As you roll under, let your weight transfer across your shoulder blades around to land in Position of Assurance.

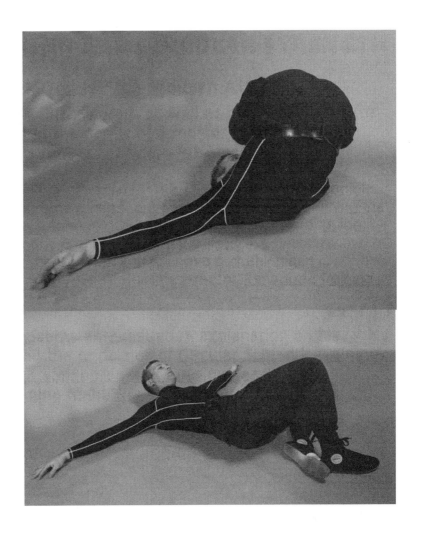

Long Arm Roll Reverse

Begin in Position of Assurance with arms outstretched to the sides.

Exhale and contract your abdomen. Do NOT throw your legs over your head! This is SLOW & CONTROLLED!

Bring your feet overhead as you move your neck in the opposite direction of your legs. Exhale!

Bend the far knee down to the ground, while placing the foot closer to your head on ball of foot.

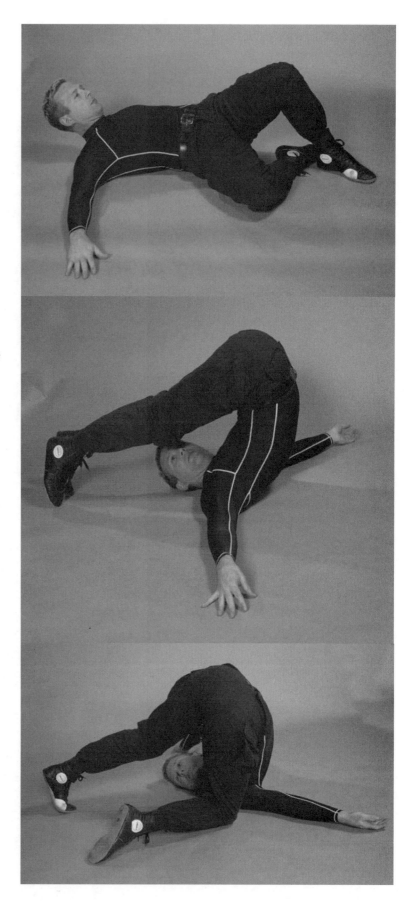

Bring the Ball of Foot close to your chest and place the entire Flat Foot down.

Simultaneously, keep tucking the far knee to land in a Shin Squat.

Unscrew your arms and arrive in the Shin Squat!

Execute the opposite Long Arm Roll and repeat the Reverse Long Arm Roll!

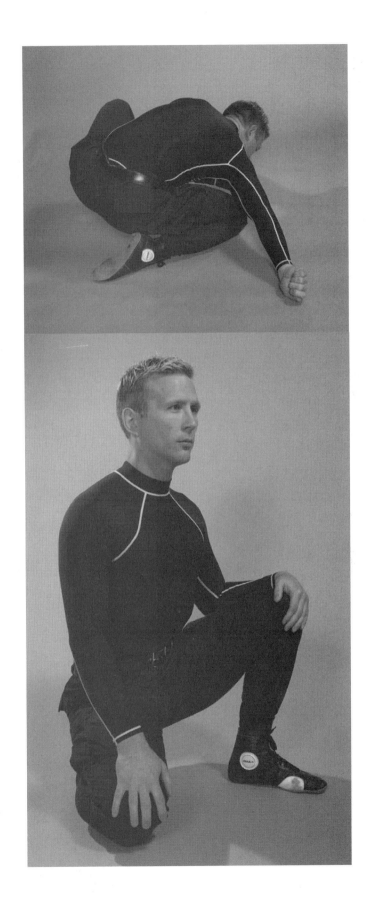

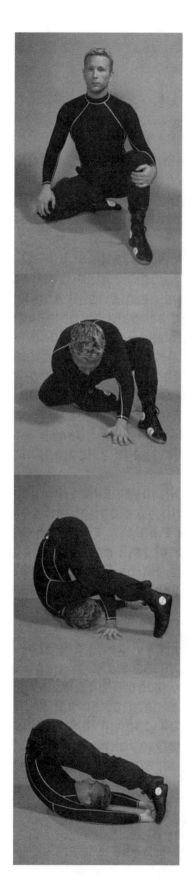

Arm Thread Shoulder Roll

Begin in Shin Squat.

Thread the arm on the same side as the planted shin between your shin and your shin and your opposite foot.

Continue to extend and screw your arm until you expose your back to the ground. You roll UNDER not over.

Use your opposite hand as a brace to guide you.

Tuck your chin and move your head under your bracing arm-pit. Your shoulder and your head should not touch the ground.

Begin your exhale.

As you roll under, lift off with the Ball of Foot of your formerly planted shin.

Exhale more deeply.

You arrive in the Spinal Rock, with legs parallel and knees slightly bent.

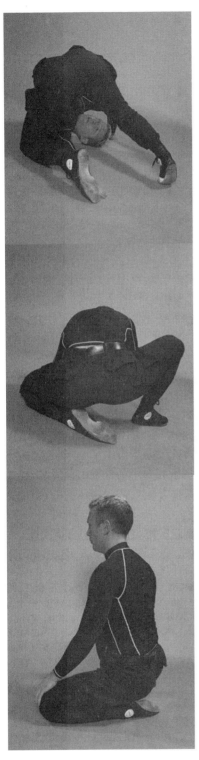

Continue the motion so that the leg that began with a Flat Foot bends at the knee to engage the ground.

Release your head in the opposite direction as you brace now with the arm that originally threaded.

Press backward and transfer your weight from your brace to your planted shin.

Allow your inhale to occur as you decompress and your chest opens again.

You arrive in the opposite Shin Squat!

Repeat and continue in a circle!

Lateral Shoulder Roll

Begin in Seated Ready.

Collapse your knee to one side softly keeping your elbow pinched to your ribs

Take your far leg and gently swing (do NOT throw your foot over!) in front of your head.

Simultaneously begin tucking your chin and allowing your head to remove underneath. There should never be any pressure on your head or neck!!!

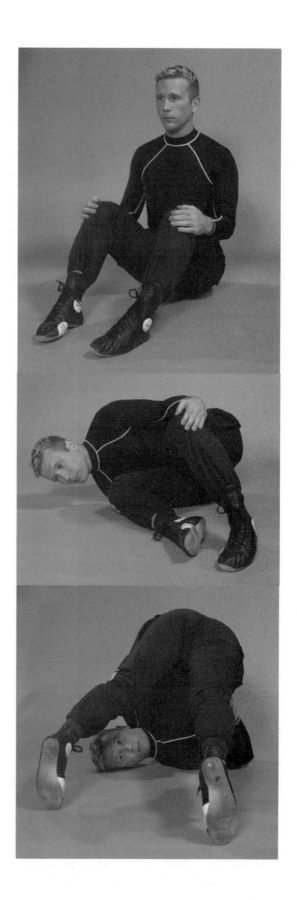

Allow your motion to continue so that you roll across the plane of your shoulder blades. Your head, neck and shoulders should feel no pressure!

You arrive in the Spinal Rock with legs parallel. You must keep your legs as far forward (over your head and touching the ground) as possible, or the momentum will take you off your shoulders and down to mid-back.

Keep the momentum thread the far knee underneath to your chest. Remember to keep the near elbow pinched to your ribs!

Transferring your weight off of your planted forearm while preserving the momentum, you arrive back in Seated Ready.

Repeat and Continue!

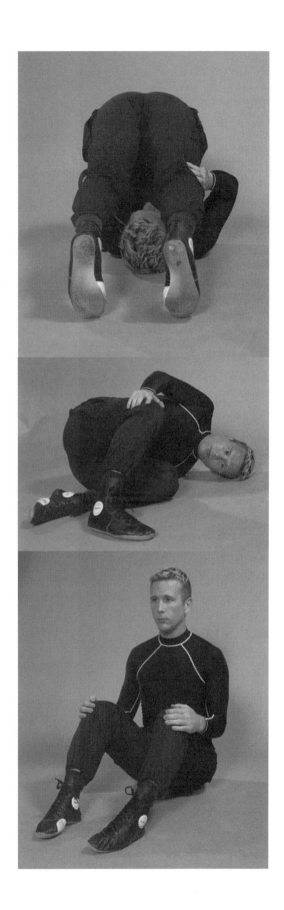

Neck Roll

Begin lying on the ground with arms outstretched.

A la Arm Screw, begin rotating one shoulder underneath you, while lifting the opposite shoulder.

Simultaneously shift your hips in the opposite direction of the elevated shoulder.

Freeing your head to travel, move it under the lifted armpit.

Exhale through the entire motion.

Contracting your abdominals and tilting your pelvis upward, continue to rotate your head underneath (a la Arm Thread Shoulder Roll.) There should never be any pressure on your neck!!!

You arrive in the Spinal Rock!

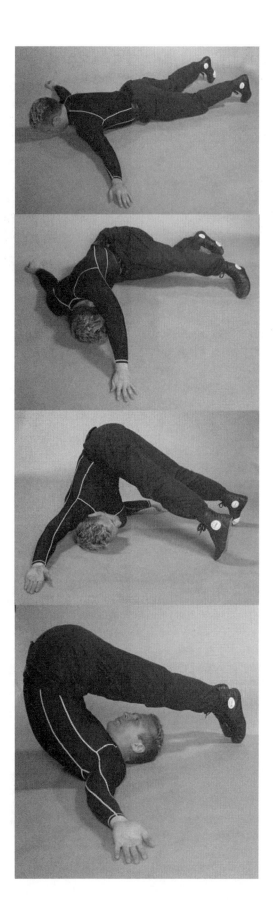

Release the
momentum in the
opposite direction by
continuing to move
your head in a circle.

Reverse your Arm
Screw and let your legs
extend, releasing your
head.

You arrive at the
beginning belly down
and arms extended to
the sides.

Repeat and continue
fluidly without pain!

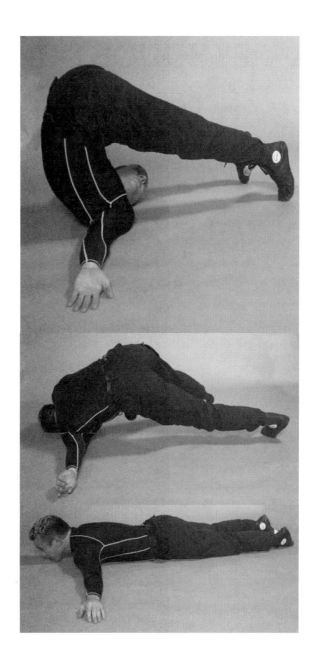

Twisting Spinal Arch

Begin in Spinal Arch with arms extended to the sides.

Slide one arm above and the other below like opposite hands of a clock.

Continue the motion allowing the higher shoulder to move over your head.

Exhale.

Maintain the momentum a la Neck Roll and arrive in the Spinal Rock structure!

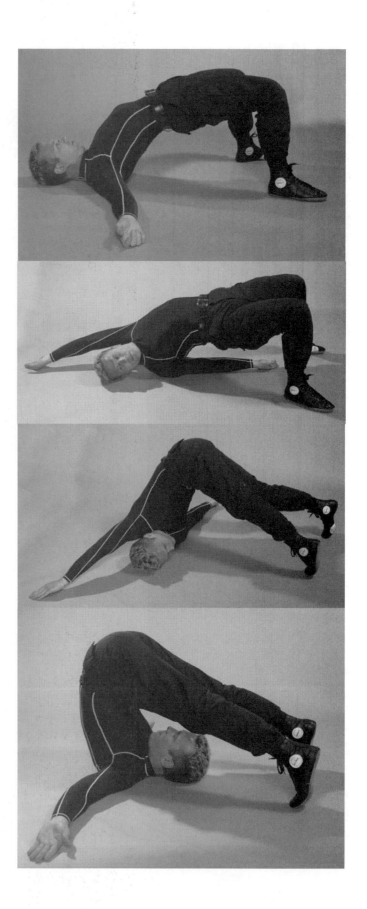

As in the Neck Roll continue to circle your head in the same direction.

However, in this exercise, continue to swing your arms in the original direction (uninterruptedly).

Keep your feet on the ground at all times!

Thread your back knee underneath while keeping your hips off of the ground.

Step through with the read leg a la Arching Leg Thread.

You arrive back in the Spinal Arch.

Repeat and Continue!

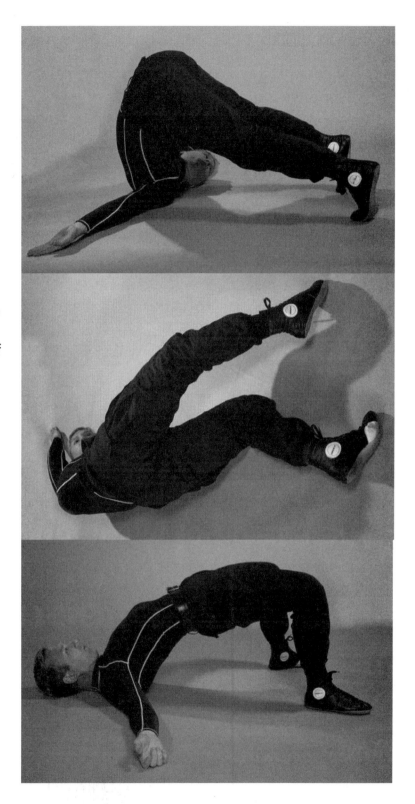

Arching High-Leg

Begin in the Spinal Rock structure. Exhale.

Bend one knee to the ground as if moving to a Shin Squat a la Long Arm Roll.

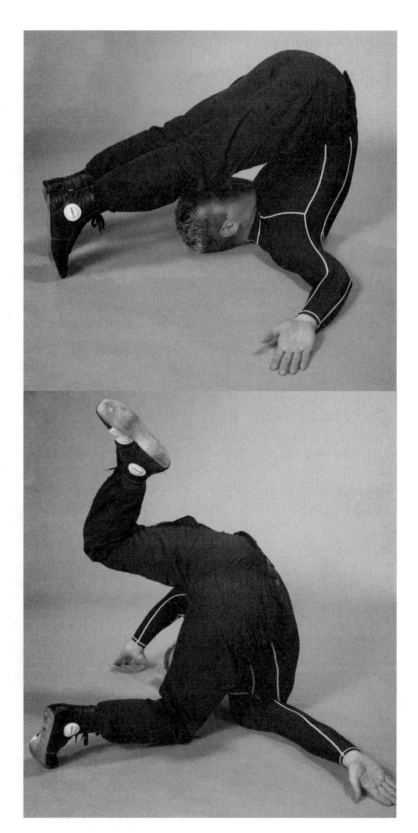

Extend your legs as in the Hurdler Stretch Spinal Rock.

Slowly extend and land in a Spinal Arch.

There should never be any pressure on your neck!

Use a Pike or Straddle Spinal Rock, an Arching Leg Thread to return to the Spinal Rock structure to Repeat and Continue!

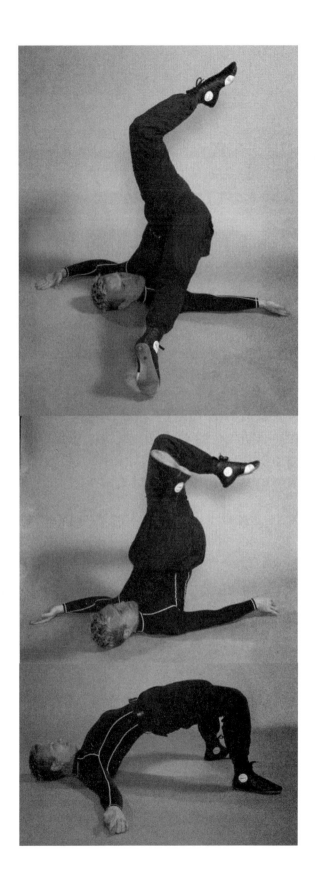

RMAX.tv PRODUCTIONS

REACHING YOUR MAXIMUM POTENTIAL

The <u>Most Trusted Source</u> in Life Enhancement since 1996

"Be more prepared than the challenges you will face!" - SCOTT SONNON, the Head Coach of the *Life Enhancement Solutions*™ Department runs a online discussion group at **RMAX.tv** where he answers questions for free and provides special offers.

Life Enhancement Solutions™ include any perceived or measurable improvement in function, in any endeavor resulting in a higher quality experience.

RMAX.tv Productions approaches Life Enhancement Solutions™ from a philosophical perspective that acknowledges each individual's right to actualize their innate talents. Regardless of where upon the spectrum of strength and skill our clients arrive with us, RMAX.tv Productions delivers unparalleled, personalized professionalism. We espouse lifetime conditioning beginning with your first step and ending with your last.

RMAX.tv Productions adopts a pioneer approach to practice, training and competition: All of our clients may receive incremental, errorless training standards. RMAX.tv Productions begins at your level and moves forward with you. RMAX emphasizes the physical, mental and spiritual development as a complete organism and creates progressive adaptations in a functional manner. RMAX.tv Productions holds the goal of preparing everyone for the physical challenges of the lifestyle in which they choose to engage.

<u>Life Enhancement</u> is the process of personal transformation through physical culture. The process holds three goals for our clients, to:

- <u>Increase Biomechanical Efficiency</u>: *the integration of breathing, movement and structural alignment.*
- <u>Decrease Fear-Reactivity</u>: *the specific behavioral patterns arising when confronted perceived threats, mistakes and unexpected events.*
- <u>Cultivate Flow-State</u>: *the peak performance experience manifesting through the attributes of exploration, improvisation, innovation.*

RMAX.tv Productions helps you cultivate three critical elements, which also comprise our institutional credo:

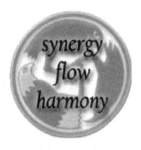

www.RMAX.tv

RMAX.tv Productions
(AARMACS, Inc)
P.O. Box 501388,
Atlanta, GA 31150, USA
Tel: 1-770-956-9765
Fax: 1-770-956-1548
info@RMAX.tv

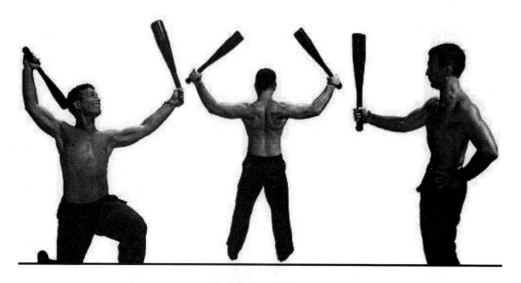

CLUBBELL TRAINING FOR CIRCULAR STRENGTH

An Ancient Tool for the Modern Athlete

Learn the exercises within this program as well as have the chance to observe Clubbell Training at the hands of a master, Coach Sonnon - the man who vitalized this fitness sensation for Americans.

"Clubbell Training for Circular Strength is a must read. Whether you're a martial artist, sports competitor, or extreme athlete, anyone will benefit from learning the information in this book. Coach Sonnon offers more than just a "how-to" guide; this book is deep in its philosophy and tradition -- it is a lifestyle, a "way." Follow Clubbell Training for Circular Strength and you will have a crushing grip ... physically, mentally, and spiritually." Grant Hansen, Director, Renegade Training International

BOOK - Coach Sonnon presents an exhaustive explanation on his Philosophy of Strength and the principles of Circular Strength Training, including how to create personal programs, design specialized programs as well as including many general strength as well as sport specific programs.

240 pages, illustrations, diagrams and photographs:

- Historical Chapter
- The Philosophy of Strength
- The Genesis of Circular Strength Training
- The Principles of Clubbell training for Circular Strength
- Strength Development Trinity
- Total Body Strength
- Rules of Clubbell Training for Circular Strength
- Clubbell Training Exercises
- Clubbell Training for Circular Strength Program Design Guidelines
- Clubbell Training for Circular Strength Program Samples
- Beginning Programs
- Strength Programs
- Endurance Programs
- Power Programs
- Advanced Programs
- Combination Routines
- Tactical & Combative Strength Programs
- Sport Specific Strength Programs
And much more...

Order clubbells and clubbells video materials at **www.Clubbell.tv**

MAX·IM·OL·O·GY

The Pursuit of Maximum Performance

Coach Sonnon's <u>Accelerated Conditioning Course for Confidence, Power, Energy, Longevity and Stamina!</u>

"Coach Sonnon is absolutely the product as advertised: knowledgeable, approachable, superlatively skilled, smart as hell, and the originator of a fascinating approach to fitness that connects the internal and external worlds of strength, fitness training and Martial Arts. He teaches our CNS [Central Nervous System], not just our muscles, and it makes all the difference in the world. I feel like my world just expanded, and that Coach Sonnon is, and I use this term with full knowledge of the risk of hyperbole, a kinesthetic genius." - Steven Barnes, former Kungfu Columnist for Black Belt Magazine, Author of <u>Lion's Blood</u>

Now YOU can access **Coach Sonnon's** personal system of ACCELERATED fitness and fighting ability, proven in champion after champion on the mat, on patrol, and on the battlefield.

Have you wanted to visit one of **Coach Sonnon's** seminars and didn't have the time to do it?
Have you wanted to enroll but none of my seminars was close to you?
Have you wanted to attend but were afraid of the commitment of the demanding certification examination?
Do you want to know how his coaching looks LIVE?
Do you want to get inside the true REALITY of his coaching as it impacts YOU?
Are you interested in finding out the TRUE nature of **Coach Sonnon's** *Circular Strength Training* system?
Do you want to get your "feet wet" without jumping in on one of **Coach Sonnon's** certification camps?

If you answered "Yes" to any of these questions, then you have this unique opportunity to experience Maximology at home personally. See **Scott Sonnon** coaching LIVE participants in a certification course in this 5 tape series. This is the ONLY seminar **Coach Sonnon** has allowed to be filmed. Do you want to take your abilities and soar high?

See RMAX.tv Productions for ordering information.

IS PROPER BREATHING NECESSARY FOR YOUR TRAINING?

The answer – YES, DEFINITELY!

Then check this videotape from Coach Sonnon:

BE BREATHED™

The Way to New Breathing - The Way to New Life

"It is not merely a program you do, but an powerful warrior you become! Don't "Just Do It" - BE IT!" - says **the creator, Coach Sonnon**.

Be Breathed™ is a revolutionary exercise program, which will enhance and integrate your breathing, movement and structural alignment.

Be Breathed™ comprises fun, low-impact programs based upon health and fitness secrets revealed for everyone.

Be Breathed™:

- Gives you healthy muscle tone and power
- Decreases your waistline
- Increases confidence in your coordination
- Increases your flexibility
- Gives you suppleness
- Magnifies your energy levels
- Increases your ability to perform daily physical tasks
- Increases your relaxation
- Gives you the ability to be calm under pressure

Be Breathed™ is a great for all ages and for the whole family, that **requires no equipment and can be done anywhere**, anytime, at home or at work, while watching television or listening to the radio, with your friends or alone, on the plane, behind the keyboard, in the car, everywhere you are!

"... Informative, easy to understand, and the demonstrations skillfully made..." -Dan Rutz, former CNN Senior Medical Correspondent

"... A viable and effective health and fitness methodology requiring no equipment...." - Marty Gallagher, Columnist for the Washington Post (washingtonpost.com), World Powerlifting Champion and Fitness Expert

Order this tape at RMAX.tv Productions, and **Be Breathed™** Every Moment of Your Life!

ZDOROVYE™

SLAVIC NATURAL HEALTH SYSTEM

ZDOROVYE – NATURE'S LEGACY™

ZDOROVYE™ is Ancient Russia's answer to Aerobic kick-boxing, Qigong, Tai-chi and Yoga combined. Zdorovye - Nature's Legacy™ is the culmination of centuries of health wisdom, and decades of scientific research in the former Soviet Union and modern Russia.

In the laboratories, physicians made amazing discoveries in the realm of Psychophysiology (the scientific discipline that view body and mind as one interrelated interdependent entity). Volumes of secrets were revealed on disease prevention, health improvement and performance enhancement. Russian Olympic and National instructors used these methods to significantly increase the health and performance of their sportsmen. The renowned, elite Special Forces of Russia (named "Spetsnaz") has also benefited from this specialized training, whereby their stamina, performance and recovery times were dramatically increased. For years, the former USSR was shrouding these health technologies in secrecy.

Finally, this revolutionary health system was translated into format understandable by the Western mind-set, by a team of American researchers, trainers and doctors, spawned and led by **Coach Sonnon**, the first foreigner permitted to train with Russian Special Forces and Olympic Trainers and certified to teach their revolutionary health and fitness secrets, which were kept in secret for many decades behind the iron curtain, and never before seen outside of Russia.

It is the effective Health System, which will benefit every single person. **Coach Sonnon** assembled this powerful system creating physical and mental wellness to improve health, prevents disease and enhance performance of daily tasks. This system re-integrates and refines Movement, Posture, and Breathing through a comprehensive process of unique, never-before-seen exercise and research. Get pain-free movement, vibrant energy, & increased longevity!

The BASIC LEVEL of Zdorovye™ comprises the 1st Trinity:

- Movement Exercise: *Dvizheniye*™ Natural Grace
- Postural Exercise: *Polozheniye*™ Natural Poise
- Breathing Exercise: *Dykhaniye*™ Natural Energy

There is also one application program available for putting Zdorovye™ in motion:

- Effortless Running called *Slavyanskiy Byeg*™ Natural Carriage

Zdorovye™ teaches that if Movement affects Posture and Breathing; Posture affects Breathing and Movement; and Breathing affects Movement and Posture. Any three characteristic negatively or positively impacts the others. Stress, trauma, anxiety or general misuse promote health decline by disintegrating your Movement, Posture, and Breathing. Zdorovye - Nature's Legacy™ is not a collection of "exercises" but a set of instruction designed to enable the individual, regardless of his or her interest, to develop a personalized style of training.

This system, if used properly, will increase the well-being of the viewer, helping the viewer to breath, stand and move with ease and in manner that improves health, prevents disease, and enhances natural performance of daily tasks (as well as extreme tasks) and ultimately makes the viewer a healthier, happier individual.

There are many applications of ZDOROVYE™. One of the most significant is sports performance enhancement because it is a scientific system of maintaining and improving health, which counters the often destructive training practices of combat sport. Zdorovye does this by increasing joint health, respiratory efficiency, soft tissue elasticity and coordination without requiring recovery, so athletes can improve their condition when they would otherwise be convalescing.

Zdorovye- Nature's Legacy™ is the next step in the evolution of the global health consciousness for the 21st century!

"…The Zdorovye system is practical in approach with straightforward techniques that are understandable on first exposure, though mastery, no doubt, takes years. All you need is a place to stand, sit or lie down. The benefits of Zdorovye training are numerous: better flexibility, improved coordination, greater joint mobility, accelerated reaction time, improved endurance, increased health, vitality and sense of well-being, refined focus and concentration. Best of all, the linked Zdorovye exercise sequence provides an all-encompassing abdominal workout that is incredibly intense and effective…" - Marty Gallagher, a World Powerlifting Champion and Fitness Expert, Washington Post Fitness Journalist.

"…No amount of written text from anyone can even come close to explaining the benefits that the Zdorovye System can have on the lives of you and your friends and family. You must experience them for yourself… " – Marc Bryan – USA Professional Fighter and Strongman

"I find they are tremendous value for athletes of all levels and can be used within many sport disciplines." - Coach John Davies, Renegade Training

WARRIOR WELLNESS™

6 Degrees of Freedom™
The ORIGINAL, the LEADER, the BEST Joint Mobility System!

Coach Sonnon Introduces his <u>Unique Joint Mobility Exercises for Joint Injury Prevention and Rehabilitation</u>.

Dynamic Range of Motion
Dynamic Relaxation
Tendon Strengthening
Joint Health and Freedom from Pain
Flexibility
Core Stability

Includes Exercise Descriptions, Program Design, and THREE Follow-Along Programs: Beginner, Intermediate and Advanced.

Coach Sonnon brings these health secrets to everyone. He developed these fun, low-impact programs that will strengthen all of the joints throughout your body, giving you confidence and coordination, healthy muscle tone and suppleness, and an energizing start to every day!

"...I have been working on a daily program for just over a week and finding my energy levels higher than usual also feeling more relaxed and fluid, whether I'm engaged in an activity or not. ... The exercises are of a progressive nature so anyone, whatever their age, skill level or condition will be able to use them immediately..." – Kon Hui Quek, Singapore

Please check **www.RMAX.tv** and **www.Clubbell.tv** for the complete product list of

<u>Life Enhancement Solutions™</u>

NOTES AND THOUGHTS

NOTES AND THOUGHTS

NOTES AND THOUGHTS

NOTES AND THOUGHTS